ATLAS OF
ESSENTIAL
PROCEDURES

ATLAS OF
ESSENTIAL
PROCEDURES

Michael Tuggy, MD

Director, Swedish Family Medicine Residency
Department of Family Medicine
University of Washington
Seattle, Washington

Jorge Garcia, MD

Associate Director, Swedish Family Medicine Residency
Department of Family Medicine
University of Washington
Seattle, Washington

ELSEVIER
SAUNDERS

1600 John F. Kennedy Blvd.
Ste 1800
Philadelphia, PA 19103-2899

ATLAS OF ESSENTIAL PROCEDURES   ISBN: 978-1-4377-1499-9

Copyright © 2011 by Saunders, an imprint of Elsevier Inc.

Notice

Knowledge and best practice in this field are constantly changing. As new research and experience broaden our knowledge, changes in practice, treatment and drug therapy may become necessary or appropriate. Readers are advised to check the most current information provided (i) on procedures featured or (ii) by the manufacturer of each product to be administered, to verify the recommended dose or formula, the method and duration of administration, and contraindications. It is the responsibility of the practitioner, relying on their own experience and knowledge of the patient, to make diagnoses, to determine dosages and the best treatment for each individual patient, and to take all appropriate safety precautions. To the fullest extent of the law, neither the Publisher nor the authors assumes any liability for any injury and/or damage to persons or property arising out of or related to any use of the material contained in this book.

The Publisher

Library of Congress Cataloging-in-Publication Data
Tuggy, Michael.
 Atlas of essential procedures / Michael Tuggy, Jorge Garcia. – 1st ed.
  p. ; cm.
 ISBN 978-1-4377-1499-9
 1. Ambulatory surgery–Handbooks, manuals, etc. I. Garcia, Jorge, 1955- II. Title.
 [DNLM: 1. Ambulatory Surgical Procedures–methods–Atlases. WO 517 T915a 2010]
 RD110.T84 2010
 617'.024–dc22

                                                                        2010011222

Editor: Kate Dimock
Developmental Editor: Taylor Ball
Publishing Services Manager: Hemamalini Rajendrababu
Project Manager: Srikumar Narayanan
Designer: Ellen Zanolle
Illustrator: Mike Carcel
Marketing Manager: Helena Mutak

Printed in China

Last digit is the print number: 9 8 7 6 5 4 3 2 1

Working together to grow
libraries in developing countries

www.elsevier.com | www.bookaid.org | www.sabre.org

ELSEVIER   BOOK AID International   Sabre Foundation

To my wife Peg, and my children, Daniel and Kristin,
thank you for your patience while I have worked on this project.

Michael Tuggy, MD

I would like to thank my brilliant and lovely wife
Dr Barbara Schinzinger, and the stellar residents and faculty
at Swedish Family Medicine Residency in Seattle.

Jorge Garcia, MD

PREFACE

The most rapid and long lasting way to learn is by engaging all the senses, especially by incorporating *visual* information. This is most clearly the case when one is trying to learn a medical procedure. For this reason, we have developed video tutorials to help achieve rapid competence in these procedures.

Additionally, *repeated* review of cognitive, visual, and manual skills can allow a learner to master and retain a procedure. For those in the medical field who need to use these procedures episodically, returning to these video tutorials will refresh and reinforce previous instruction.

It is increasingly recognized that *standardization* of procedures can lead to improved safety. We hope that learners will apply these standard methods as shown in the video and text so that we can offer procedures to our patients that are safe and produce the desired outcome.

As medical educators, we have found that by using these video tutorials we achieve learning *efficiency* that was not possible with only pictures and text. We have used these videos to teach and test competency in medical procedures.

Come back to this text often to review and relearn.

Michael Tuggy, MD

Jorge Garcia, MD

ACKNOWLEDGMENT

We offer our sincere gratitude to our patients, who allowed us to use images of themselves undergoing the procedures in this text, and to our future patients, who will be better served by the generosity of others whom they will never know.

CONTENTS

Dermatology

Chapter 1

Punch Biopsy

COMMON INDICATIONS

Punch biopsy is a good choice for the complete removal of small lesions (less than 5 mm) and for the pathologic diagnosis of a larger lesion (Figure 1-1).

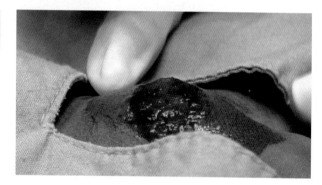

FIGURE 1-1. Punch biopsy is useful in obtaining a pathologic specimen of skin lesions.

EQUIPMENT

A punch biopsy instrument used to obtain a full-thickness cylindrical specimen is added to the routine skin repair set that includes a topical anesthetic such as 1% lidocaine, pick-ups or forceps, iris scissors, and a labeled specimen cup (Figure 1-2).

KEY STEPS

1. **Prepare the lesion:** Place the patient in a comfortable position that allows adequate access to the area to be biopsied. Prepare the selected site with alcohol or povidone iodine. Use a sterile technique if sutures are intended.

2. **Topical anesthesia:** Place a ring of anesthesia around the lesion (infiltration block) or deep to the lesion, depending on the size (Figure 1-3).

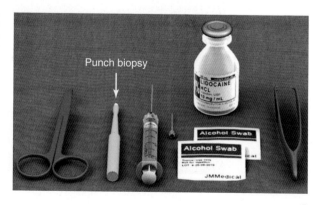

FIGURE 1-2. Equipment includes the punch biopsy and skin repair kit.

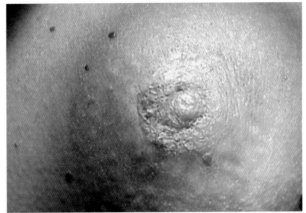

FIGURE 1-3. Anesthetize the area with 1% lidocaine.

3. **Punch biopsy:** Choose the appropriate sized punch instrument (2 to 5 mm). To minimize scarring, stretch the skin on both sides of the planned biopsy site away from the site, perpendicular to the lines of minimal skin tension, using the thumb and index finger of the nondominant hand (Figure 1-4). Gently push the punch instrument vertically into the skin and rotate it to cut through the skin to the subcutaneous fat. A decrease in resistance should be felt at the point where the dermis is completely penetrated (Figure 1-5). Withdraw the punch. Push down with the fingers on each side of the biopsy. If the "plug" goes down with the skin, the biopsy has not gone deep enough. If the plug pops up instead of going down, then the adipose tissue has been entered, and the tissue has been freed adequately. Gently grasp the specimen with forceps or a skin hook. Lift the specimen, and free it by cutting the subcutaneous base with sharp tissue scissors (Figure 1-6).

4. **Hemostasis:** Apply pressure for hemostasis. Biopsies of 2 or 3 mm do not need to be closed with sutures. A 4-mm punch biopsy on the face may need to be sutured, and a 5-mm punch biopsy nearly always requires suturing.

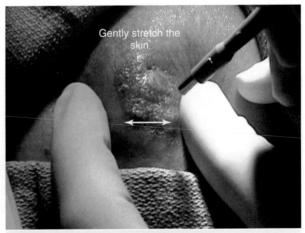

FIGURE 1-4. Gently stretch the skin.

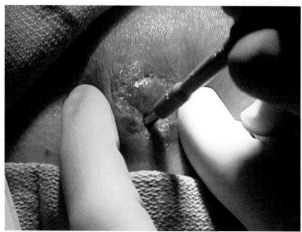

FIGURE 1-5. Rotate the punch instrument through to the subcutaneous fat.

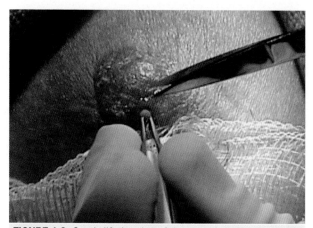

FIGURE 1-6. Gently lift the plug of tissue and cut the base with scissors.

ICD-9 CODES

173.9   Skin neoplasm, primary malignant
198.2   Skin neoplasm, secondary malignant
232.9   Skin neoplasm, carcinoma in situ
216.9   Skin neoplasm, benign
238.2   Skin neoplasm, uncertain behavior
239.2   Skin neoplasm, unspecified

Chapter 2

Shave Biopsy

COMMON INDICATION

A shave biopsy is used to remove the protruding portion of a raised skin lesion when a full-thickness sample is not required. Advantages of a shave excision include a minimal time requirement, simple equipment, and the lack of need for reapproximation and suturing, and generally good cosmetic results (Figure 2-1).

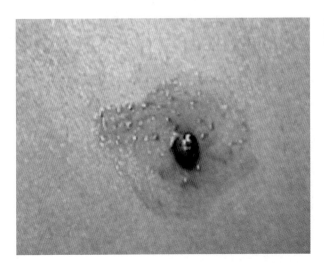

FIGURE 2-1. A shave biopsy is used to remove the protruding portion of a raised skin lesion.

EQUIPMENT

Volumes of 0.5 to 1.0 cc of 1% to 2% lidocaine, with or without epinephrine, are generally used for local anesthesia. Draw up the anesthetic with an 18-gauge needle, and then use a 27- or 30-gauge needle for injection. Use a 15 blade scalpel, a single double-edged razor blade, or a radiofrequency unit for shave biopsies (Figure 2-2).

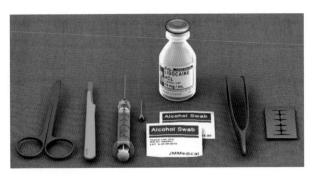

FIGURE 2-2. Equipment.

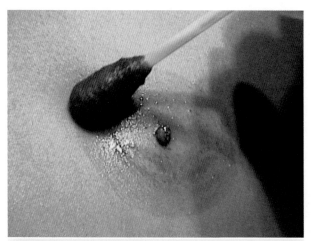

FIGURE 2-3. Prepare the skin.

KEY STEPS

1. **Position patient:** Place the patient in a position that is comfortable for him or her and still allows adequate access to the area to be biopsied. Shave excisions should not be performed if a melanoma is suspected because it may interfere with the pathologist's ability to grade the depth of the invasion.

2. **Prepare lesion:** Prepare the area with povidone iodine or alcohol, and use a clean technique; sterile gloves are not necessary (Figure 2-3).

3. **Anesthesia:** Instill a local anesthetic within the dermis underneath the lesion to slightly elevate the lesion (Figure 2-4).

Scalpel Technique

1. **Lesion excision:** Excise the lesion by shaving with a scalpel blade kept parallel to the skin (Figure 2-5).

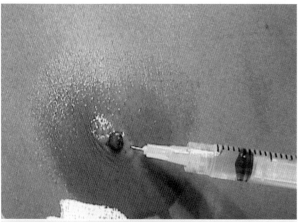

FIGURE 2-4. Anesthetize the lesion.

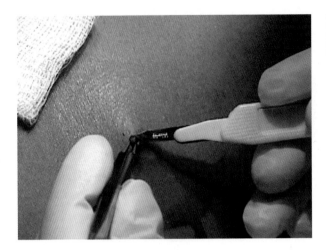

FIGURE 2-5. Scalpel excision, keeping the blade parallel to the skin.

2. **Wound care:** After shaving the lesion, apply simple pressure and pinpoint electrodesiccation, radiofrequency coagulation or a topical agent, such as aluminum chloride, or Monsel's solution to achieve hemostasis (Figure 2-6).

Razor Blade Technique

Lesion excision: Pick-ups can be used to gently bow the blade toward the lesion. Removal is accomplished by gently rocking the razor blade against the base of the lesion (Figure 2-7).

Radiofrequency Technique

1. **Lesion excision:** Shave excision can be performed using a radiofrequency loop (Figure 2-8). Heat artifact may occur at the margin of the excision, hindering histopathologic evaluation, or, in the case of a very thin lesion, obliterating the lesion entirely. Also, because of the ease of cutting with a radiofrequency loop, the novice user may inadvertently go too deep with the loop, causing excessive and unnecessary scarring.

2. **Wound repair:** Many practitioners perform a shave biopsy with a scalpel blade and use a radiofrequency loop to feather out the edge of the defect created to complete the procedure (Figure 2-9).

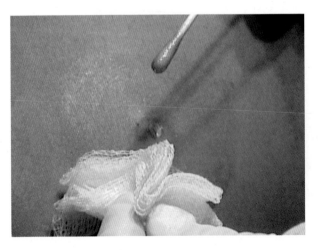

FIGURE 2-6. Achieve hemostasis with pressure or with Monsel's solution.

FIGURE 2-7. Razor blade excision, using a rocking motion.

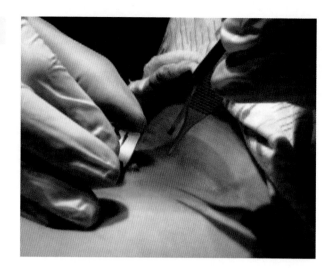

FIGURE 2-8. Radiofrequency excision, using care to avoid excess depth.

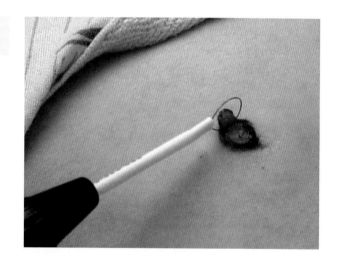

FIGURE 2-9. Radiofrequency to remove lesion edges.

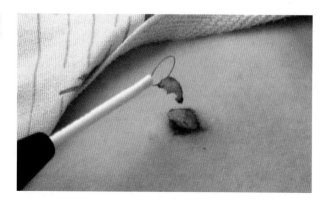

ICD-9 CODES

173.9   Skin neoplasm, primary malignant
198.2   Skin neoplasm, secondary malignant
232.9   Skin neoplasm, carcinoma in situ
216.9   Skin neoplasm, benign
238.2   Skin neoplasm, uncertain behavior
239.2   Skin neoplasm, unspecified

Chapter 3

Excisional Biopsy

COMMON INDICATION

Excisional biopsies are most often performed using an elliptical excision around a skin lesion, followed by a full-depth removal of the lesion with a surrounding margin of normal skin (Figure 3-1).

EQUIPMENT

The minimum equipment needed for an excisional biopsy includes a needle driver, iris scissors, Adson's forceps, a No. 15 blade scalpel, and a curved hemostat (Figure 3-2). A variety of sutures are used for closure, depending on the location of the biopsy and the wound tension. Generally, a 4-O nylon suture will provide adequate wound closure for most areas. If a subcuticular closure is planned, use a 3-O or 4-O absorbable braided suture.

KEY STEPS

1. **Anesthesia:** Cleanse the skin with alcohol, and inject local anesthetic in a field block around the planned ellipse of the incision. Ensure that the local block is wide enough for the incision and for undermining the skin edges (Figure 3-3). After the block is placed, cleanse the skin with Betadine then drape the area to create a sterile field.

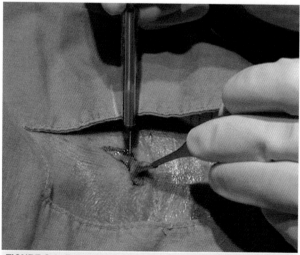

FIGURE 3-1. Full-depth skin lesions removed with an excisional biopsy.

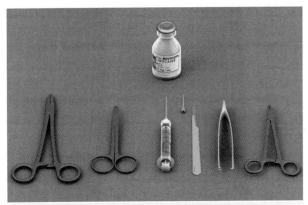

FIGURE 3-2. Equipment for excisional biopsy.

2. **Incision:** The longitudinal axis of the elliptical excision should follow the skin lines (Figure 3-4). The skin is excised fully through the dermis to obtain a full thickness biopsy. Once the ellipse is created, the tissue sample is completely removed by severing the underlying subcutaneous attachments. Use short strokes with the No. 15 blade scalpel to incise down to the subcutaneous fat layer.

3. **Undermining:** To reduce the tension on the wound while it is healing, undermine the dermis along the lateral margins of the excision. Use iris scissors to undermine the margins at least 0.5 cm and larger for higher tension wounds (Figure 3-5).

4. **Deep closure:** If the incision is large enough and deep tissue layers have adequate tensile strength, then a deep layer of absorbable suture may be used to reduce wound tension and can also control bleeding if present in the deeper layer. Usually two or three deep stitches are adequate to support the closure of small excisions. In this case, a single-layer closure is performed with the needle passing through the subcutaneous layer to close that layer with the skin surface and dermis.

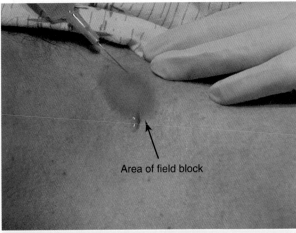

Area of field block

FIGURE 3-3. Area of field block anesthesia.

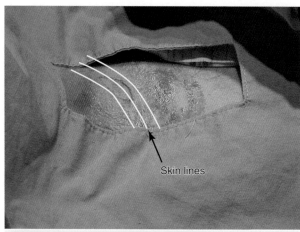

FIGURE 3-4. Cut ellipse long axis follows skin lines.

5. **Skin closure:** Simple interrupted sutures are placed to bring the wound edges together to allow healing with minimal scarring. Evert the skin edges when passing the needle perpendicularly through the skin (Figure 3-6). Place the stitches 2 to 4 mm apart, depending on the thickness of the skin. For thin skin and a fine suture, place the sutures 2 to 3 mm apart. For thicker skin and less cosmetically sensitive areas, spacing the sutures 3 to 4 mm apart will allow for good closure. Increase the density of the sutures when closing high-tension areas (Figure 3-7). Perform instrument ties with four throws in each stitch to keep the stitch from unraveling. The first knot should be a surgeon's knot to prevent it from slipping. Cut the sutures short at 3 to 4 mm lengths.

6. **Aftercare:** After closure, cover the wound with a dressing, and have the patient return in 5 to 10 days for suture removal, depending on the wound site. Facial wounds will need sutures in place for 5 days, whereas distal extremity wounds require sutures to be in place for 8 to 10 days. Wound care and follow-up instructions should be provided to every patient.

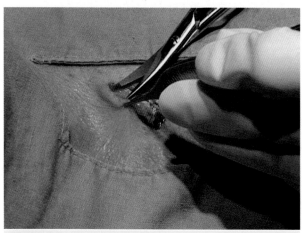

FIGURE 3-5. Undermine the dermis.

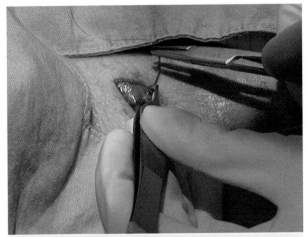

FIGURE 3-6. Everting skin to place a suture.

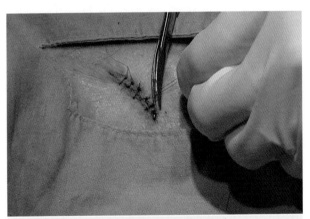

FIGURE 3-7. Suture spacing based on the tension and thickness of the skin.

ICD-9 CODES

No ICD-9 codes are associated with this procedure.

Chapter 4

Curettage and Cautery

COMMON INDICATIONS

Curettage and cautery is an effective technique for eradicating superficial basal cell carcinomas and benign superficial skin lesions such as molluscum contagiosum. Suspicious lesions can be confirmed with either a shave biopsy or a punch biopsy before the procedure, or a shave biopsy can be performed as the first step of the curettage and cautery procedure. This procedure should not be done for lesions that have advanced through the dermis (Figure 4-1).

EQUIPMENT

The equipment consists of a surgical marker, a skin curette, and an electrosurgical device that is capable of cautery. Either a ball tip electrode or a blunt tip electrode is used for the cautery phases (Figure 4-2).

KEY STEPS

1. The lesion is marked with a surgical marker to clearly delineate the extent of the superficial cancer.
2. Local anesthesia consisting of lidocaine with epinephrine is infiltrated under the lesion (Figure 4-3).
3. Use the curette to scrape the lesion from the skin surface and down into the dermal layer (Figure 4-4).

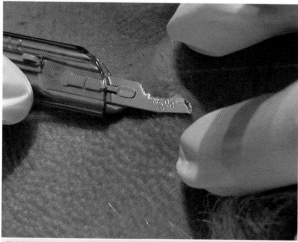

FIGURE 4-1. Shave biopsy as first step of curettage and cautery.

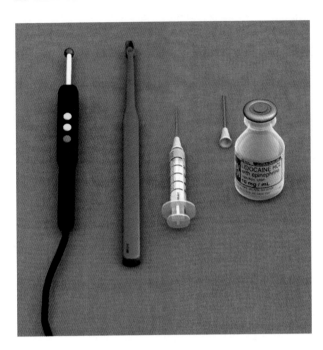

FIGURE 4-2. Equipment.

4. The lesion is curetted in four directions, with cautery being performed with each series of curettage (Figure 4-5).

5. As curettage is performed, the operator should be able to sense the softness of the basal cell cancer in contrast to the normal dermal layer. All areas of abnormal density tissue will need to be removed in the process.

6. Four rounds of curettage and cautery are performed to ensure that the process eradicates any superficial dermal extension of the basal cell cancer (Figure 4-6).

7. The wound is covered with a simple adhesive bandage upon completion of the procedure. Inspect the site at 6 months to ensure that no tumor has recurred.

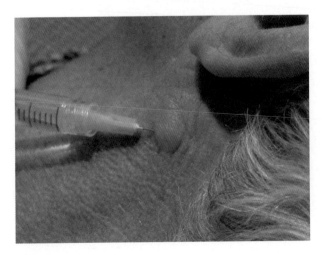

FIGURE 4-3. Local anesthesia infiltration.

FIGURE 4-4. Curettage performed in four directions.

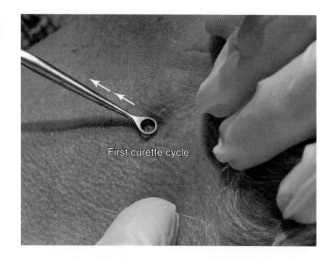

First curette cycle

FIGURE 4-5. Fourth cycle of curettage in clockwise rotation through the lesion.

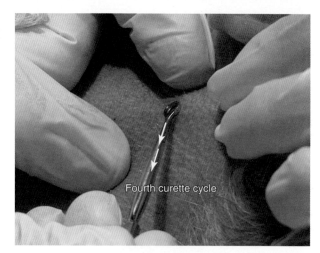

Fourth curette cycle

FIGURE 4-6. Application of cautery after each cycle to eradicate basal cell extensions.

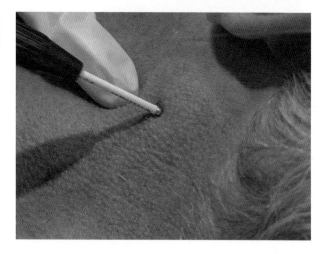

ICD-9 CODES

173.9   Skin neoplasm, primary malignant
198.2   Skin neoplasm, secondary malignant
232.9   Skin neoplasm, carcinoma in situ
216.9   Skin neoplasm, benign
238.2   Skin neoplasm, uncertain behavior
239.2   Skin neoplasm, unspecified

Chapter 5

Cryosurgery

COMMON INDICATIONS

Cryotherapy can be an effective and rapid treatment for a variety of skin lesions, including common warts, seborrheic keratosis, and actinic keratosis (Figure 5-1).

KEY STEPS

1. **Clean lesions:** Cryotherapy typically uses liquid nitrogen applied with a cotton-tipped applicator or a cryogun spray unit. The skin should be clean, but a topical anesthetic is not normally necessary.

2. **Pare wart to decrease size:** Often the efficacy of cryotherapy can be improved by paring down the wart to the level of the skin before freezing.

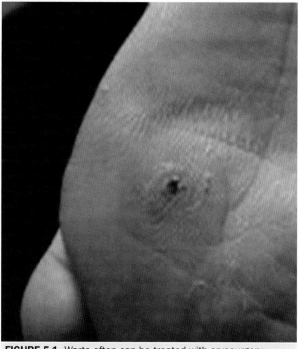

FIGURE 5-1. Warts often can be treated with cryosurgery.

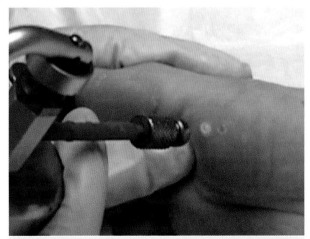

FIGURE 5-2. Freeze 2 to 3 mm beyond the edge of the wart.

3. **First freeze:** Spray each lesion (in this case, warts) with liquid nitrogen. Freeze the entire lesion, and create a 1- to 2-mm margin of white beyond the edge of the lesion. A series of lesions can be frozen in succession. Allow the frozen lesion to thaw completely, and then refreeze it (Figure 5-2).

4. **Second freeze:** The double-freeze cycle increases the efficacy of cryotherapy treatment (Figure 5-3). The patient may need to return to have the lesions treated a second or third time (Figure 5-4).

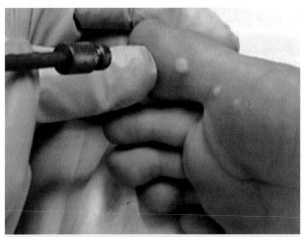

FIGURE 5-3. Double-freeze technique increases the efficacy of treatment.

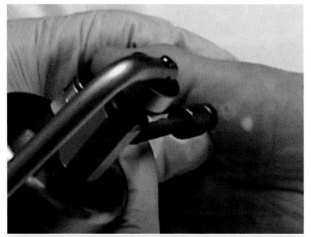

FIGURE 5-4. A second treatment in 2 to 4 weeks may be necessary.

ICD-9 CODES

No ICD-9 codes are associated with this procedure.

Chapter 6

Abscess Incision and Drainage

COMMON INDICATIONS

An abscess is a localized infection characterized by a collection of pus surrounded by inflamed tissue. A small abscess may respond to warm compresses or antibiotics and drain spontaneously. However, the treatment of choice for an abscess is incision and drainage (I & D). If this treatment is done properly, antibiotics are usually unnecessary.

EQUIPMENT

A local anesthetic, such as 1% to 2% lidocaine, is used for this procedure. A syringe with a 25- to 30-gauge needle, usually ½ to 1 in., is ideal because only the skin over the abscess is anesthetized. Other materials include an alcohol or povidone-iodine wipe, 4×4-in. gauze, No. 11 or 15 blade, curved hemostats, packing gauze, and, possibly, culture materials (Figure 6-1).

KEY STEPS

1. **Prepare skin:** Prepare the abscess area with povidone-iodine or alcohol. Carefully palpate the abscess to accurately determine the size and location (Figure 6-2). Use protective eyewear. Purulent material can "squirt out" if pressure is applied.

2. **Field block anesthesia:** Administer a field block with a local anesthetic to allow an adequate incision. Avoid infiltration of the abscess cavity (Figure 6-3). Concentrate on anesthetizing the perimeter of the tissue around the abscess. Local anesthetics are less effective in the acidic milieu of an abscess. More anesthetic than usual may be needed to relieve pain.

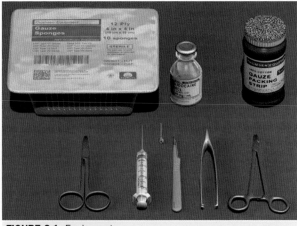

FIGURE 6-1. Equipment.

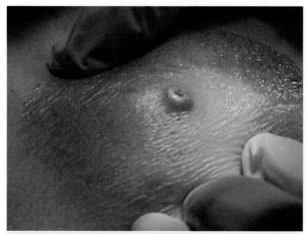

FIGURE 6-2. Gently palpate the abscess.

3. **Incision of abscess:** Make an incision with a scalpel blade to allow drainage of the abscess cavity and to prevent premature closure of the incision (Figure 6-4). When possible, make the incision along the skin lines.

4. **Drain pus:** Apply gentle external pressure to express all of the pus (Figure 6-5). Thoroughly explore the abscess cavity with a sterile cotton-tipped applicator or with hemostats. Attempts should be made to break down any walled-off pockets or possible septa (Figure 6-6).

5. **Pack cavity:** Pack the cavity with packing material, preferably iodoform gauze (Figure 6-7). The length and width used for the packing depends on the abscess size. After packing the wound, leave a small "tail" of gauze protruding from the wound to allow for drainage and eventual removal of the gauze. Apply an ointment over the wound to prevent the packing gauze from sticking to the overlying dressing, which can lead to an accidental removal of the packing when the dressing is changed.

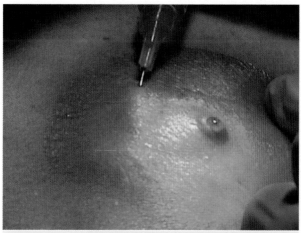

FIGURE 6-3. Inject anesthetic to create a field block.

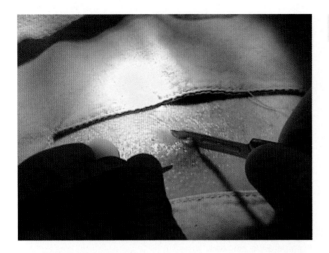

FIGURE 6-4. Incise into abscess cavity.

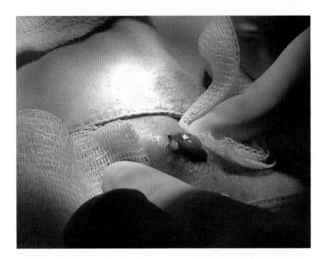

FIGURE 6-5. Gently express pus.

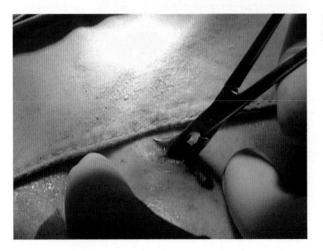

FIGURE 6-6. Explore the abscess cavity with hemostat.

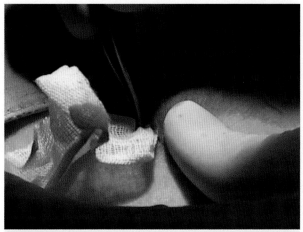

FIGURE 6-7. Pack the cavity with gauze.

ICD-9 CODES

For ICD-9-CM diagnostic codes, look under "abscess" for specific site.

Chapter 7

Wart Treatment

COMMON INDICATIONS

Patients frequently request the removal of warts to decrease discomfort and for cosmetic concerns (Figure 7-1).

KEY STEPS

Warts can be treated with a variety of methods, such as electrocautery and cryotherapy. Electrocautery is one of the most effective techniques for plantar warts, but careful attention is needed to avoid scarring.

Electrocautery and Curettage

1. **Anesthesia:** All lesions must be cleaned and locally anesthetized. Gently infiltrate 1 to 2 cc of 1% lidocaine under the lesion (Figure 7-2).

2. **Debulk the lesion:** If necessary, excise the bulk of large warts with a scalpel blade before electrocautery (Figure 7-3). Plantar warts can then be moistened with sterile water to improve the keratin response to electrodessication.

3. **Electrocautery:** With the electrocautery unit set on fulguration, lightly touch the wart for 2 to 3 seconds (Figure 7-4).

4. **Curettage:** After electrocautery, gently but thoroughly pare away the lesion with a curette (Figure 7-5). Repeat the cycle of light and brief electrocautery, alternating with curettage until the lesion is removed. Carefully control the depth of treatment of plantar warts with electrocautery and curettage. Excessive treatment can promote painful scarring. Treat bleeding, if necessary, with gentle pressure, and cover the lesion with a bandage.

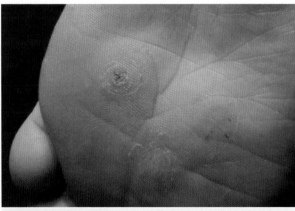

FIGURE 7-1. Plantar wart.

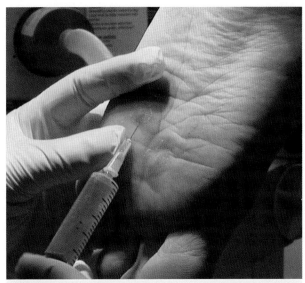

FIGURE 7-2. Anesthesia.

Cryotherapy

1. **No anesthesia required:** Liquid nitrogen cryotherapy can be an effective initial approach to common and plantar warts. Usually no anesthesia is necessary.

2. **First freeze:** Using the cryogun, aim a stream of liquid nitrogen at the center of the wart, and allow the ice ball to expand outward to include the entire lesion (Figure 7-6). Usually 3 to 5 seconds or less is sufficient to freeze the lesion.

3. **Second freeze:** A second application of nitrogen can be used after the ice has fully melted (Figure 7-7). Avoid excessive treatment of plantar warts. All modalities, including cryotherapy, can promote painful scarring.

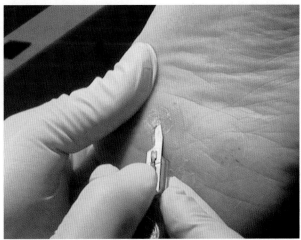

FIGURE 7-3. Scalpel excision.

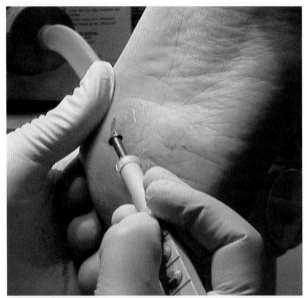

FIGURE 7-4. Electrocautery.

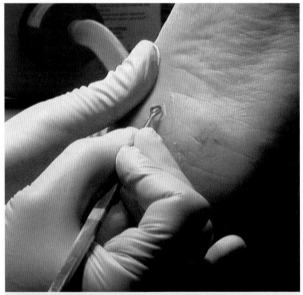

FIGURE 7-5. Curettage.

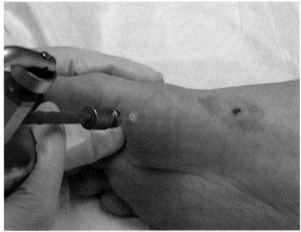

FIGURE 7-6. Cryogun first freeze.

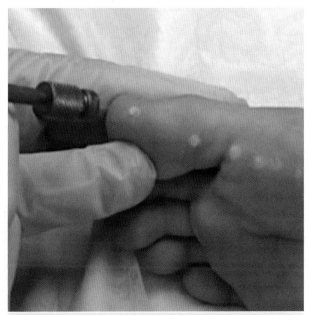

FIGURE 7-7. Cryogun second freeze.

ICD-9 CODES

07810   Verruca vulgaris (all presentations)

Chapter 8

Local Anesthesia Injection

COMMON INDICATIONS

Local anesthesia is administered with three different methods when attempting to provide patients with complete anesthesia for minor skin surgery. These include local infiltration, field block, and digital block. Select an appropriate anesthetic based on the site of the procedure, the length of desired anesthesia, and the circulatory status of the site. Never use anesthetics with vasoconstrictive agents, such as epinephrine, for digital blocks, penile blocks, or in areas of poor vascular redundancy such as the tip of the nose or the pinna of the ear (Figure 8-1).

EQUIPMENT

Draw up the anesthetic with a volume sufficient to infiltrate the procedure site. Usually 1 to 5 cc is adequate, depending on the procedure. Buffering the anesthetic with one-third dilution of sodium bicarbonate can substantially reduce the pain of injection. Use an 18-gauge needle to draw up the anesthetic, then switch to a 25- to 30-gauge needle for the injection (Figure 8-2). The injection can be done with clean gloves before the final cleansing and draping of the skin when sterility must be maintained.

Consider the use of long-acting anesthetics in areas where a prolonged block is not going to significantly affect the patient's function. Using long-acting agents versus using a short-acting agent alone significantly reduces post-procedure pain by better modulating the pain response.

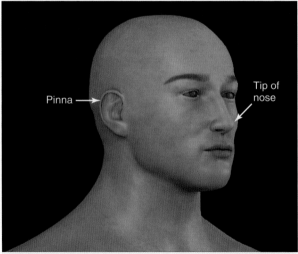

FIGURE 8-1. Examples of anatomic areas of poor vascular flow.

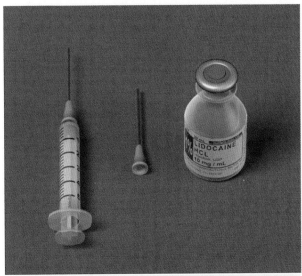

FIGURE 8-2. Equipment.

KEY STEPS

1. **Local infiltration:** Cleanse the area to be injected with alcohol or other antiseptic solution. Insert the needle at least 3 mm from the desired anesthetic area, if doing a deep infiltration for a larger infiltration block. Stepping back the site from the margin of the desired block ensures that the local block fully encompasses the area on the proximal aspect of the injection area. For small areas, such as skin wheals, insert the needle into the dermis at the edge of the desired block. Inject the anesthetic either in the dermis or in the subcutaneous layer, repositioning as needed to achieve adequate infiltration (Figure 8-3).

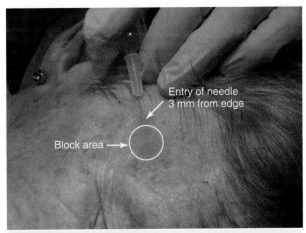

FIGURE 8-3. Local infiltration.

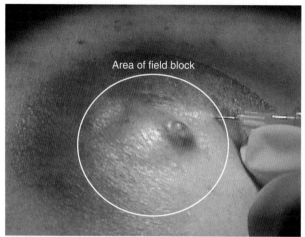

FIGURE 8-4. Field block.

2. **Field block:** Use a 1½-in. 25- or 27-gauge needle to perform the field block. This block is ideal for larger excisions where undermining is anticipated to reduce the closure tension. Inject the anesthetic in a diamond-shaped pattern that starts beyond the apices of the planned incision. Insert the needle just under the dermis, and advance the needle to the fullest extent needed. Inject while withdrawing the needle. Withdraw the needle, and repeat the injection along the adjacent line of the diamond pattern that makes up the field block. Repeat on the opposite side of the field. For a larger excision or a deep excision of masses, infiltrate under the center of the field area below the lesion or mass to be excised. This ensures that the deep layers will be adequately anesthetized. Test the planned incision line, and inject directly along that line if the lateral injections fail to fully anesthetize the center area of the diamond (Figure 8-4).

3. **Digital block:** Draw up 3 to 5 cc of anesthetic into a syringe. Cleanse the base and intertriginous areas of the digit to be blocked. Inject 0.5 to 1 cc of anesthetic at 2 o'clock and 10 o'clock positions to block the dorsal digital nerves. After 1 minute, pass the needle down from the previous injection sites to the 8 o'clock and 4 o'clock positions, and inject similar amounts of anesthetic and block the palmar or plantar nerves. For large digits, such as the great toe, the block may take as long as 10 minutes to fully take effect. Always aspirate before injecting to ensure that direct arterial injection of the anesthetic does not occur. Using a moderately tightened tourniquet can improve the duration of a digital block and reduce bleeding during a procedure. It is most useful for procedures that involve fingers and should not be left on longer than 30 minutes (Figure 8-5).

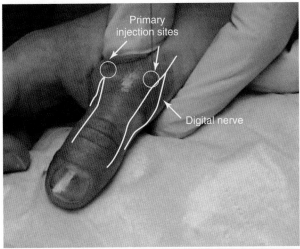

FIGURE 8-5. Digital block.

ICD-9 CODES

V14.4   Anesthetic agent

968.9   Other and unspecified local anesthetics

E855.2   Local anesthetics

Chapter 9

Electrosurgery

COMMON INDICATIONS

Electrosurgery is a powerful method in performing medically necessary and cosmetic skin procedures in the office setting. The most common cases involve the removal of moles and spider veins, or telangiectasias (Figure 9-1).

EQUIPMENT

A radiofrequency or electrocautery device provides a wide variety of common clinical uses. In the outpatient setting, mole removal, spider vein ablation, and telangiectasia ablation are useful skills. There are multiple devices on the market with similar uses, although the technology differences may provide different effects when the tools are used. The device has a variety of tips; straight wire, loops, and ball tips are needed for these procedures (Figure 9-2). To assist in identifying the margins of the mole, a surgical marker can be used to highlight the lesion to be removed. This is especially useful for flat nevi, where the margins are not elevated.

KEY STEPS

Cosmetic Mole Removal

1. **Loop technique:** Place a local block under the lesion, and wipe the lesion with alcohol to keep it moistened. The block should be placed below the dermis to prevent distortion of the junction between the nevus and the surrounding dermal layer.

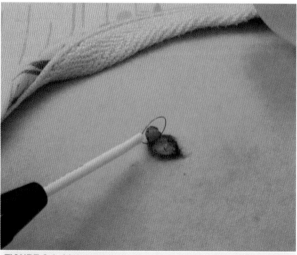

FIGURE 9-1. Mole removal.

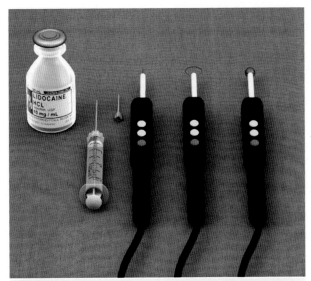

FIGURE 9-2. Local anesthetic equipment with fine wire, loop, and ball-tip attachments.

2. Use the ¼-in. loop tip on the radiofrequency scalpel to carefully excise the mole to the dermis. For the initial passes, the CUT mode is used for the removal of the bulk of the mole. For the fine passes near the base, the device can be switched to the CUT/COAG mode to provide fine coagulation for hemostasis. The loop pencil is handled very lightly to avoid excessive depth of excision. Use a light brushing stroke to remove the mole layer by layer (Figure 9-3).

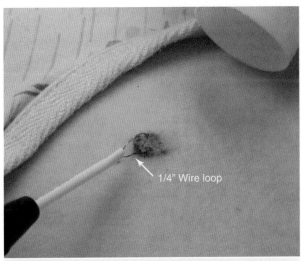

FIGURE 9-3. Mole removal with brushing stroke using a ¼-in. loop.

3. **Loop-and-ball technique:** The second stage involves the removal of a forehead lesion that is well demarcated at its base so a surgical marker is not used. The local block has been placed and is visible by the blanching of the skin around the base of the nevus. Again, use the ¼-in. loop tip on the radiofrequency scalpel to carefully shave the mole to the dermis. For the initial passes, the CUT mode is used for the removal of the bulk of the mole. Initially shave off 1 to 2 mm of depth at a time, then begin to make even thinner cuts as the base of the nevus is approached (Figure 9-4, A). (When only a small remnant of the nevus is left behind, the tip of the pencil is switched to the small ball-tip to lightly coagulate the remnants of the mole rim. After each layer is coagulated, firmly wipe the area with gauze, which removes the layer that was just coagulated. After repeating the procedure three to four times, the nevus will be fully eradicated, and only the surface of the dermis remains. Perform one final coagulation of the base of the lesion for hemostasis (Figure 9-4, B).

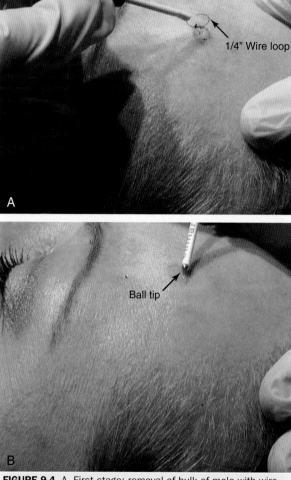

FIGURE 9-4. A. First stage: removal of bulk of mole with wire loop. B. Second stage: ablation of base of mole with ball tip.

Spider Vein Ablation

1. Place the patient in a comfortable position with the spider veins exposed. Cleanse the skin overlying the veins with an alcohol wipe. Set the device to the COAG setting, at the lowest power setting needed to pass through the skin. At this power level, no anesthesia is required. The patient will feel a small pinching sensation with each activation of the instrument.

2. Place the fine wire tip relatively perpendicular to the skin surface over the vein. Apply slight pressure with the fine wire tip on the overlying skin. Activate the device using the blue COAG button, preferably with the foot pedal to avoid movement of the hand. Upon activation, the fine tip dives through the dermis into the vein, inducing coagulation of the vein. Whenever possible, ablate junctions where the veins first branch, then repeat ablations along any remaining veins that are still visible (Figure 9-5).

3. Often two to three coagulations are required to ablate moderate-sized spider veins. For larger complexes of veins, as in this patient, 10 to 15 passes may be needed to eradicate the full complex. With larger veins, immediate blanching will occur, but maximal fading of the veins will occur 1 to 2 weeks after the procedure.

Telangiectasias

1. Place the patient in a comfortable position with the telangiectasia exposed. Cleanse the skin overlying the area with an alcohol wipe. Set the device to the COAG setting, at a low power. At this power level, no anesthesia is required. The patient will feel a small pinching sensation with every activation of the instrument, but it is well tolerated.

2. Place the fine wire tip relatively perpendicular to the skin surface over the central vein of the telangiectasia. Apply slight pressure with the fine wire tip on the overlying skin. Activate the device using the blue COAG button, preferably with the foot pedal to avoid movement of the hand. Upon activation, the fine tip dives through the dermis into the vein, inducing coagulation of the vein. When the central vein is

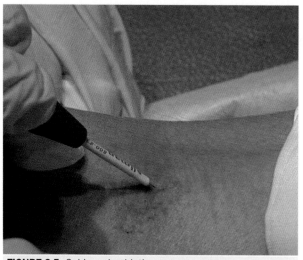

FIGURE 9-5. Spider vein ablation.

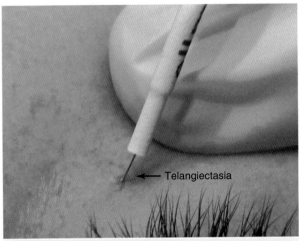

FIGURE 9-6. Ablation of telangiectasia.

ablated, re-treat any areas where there are any veins that did not coagulate immediately (Figure 9-6).

3. The results are immediate, and the patient does not need any special wound care.

ICD-9 CODES

Billing codes are based on the procedure (see notes under CPT Codes).

CPT CODES

Billing codes for radiofrequency surgery are diverse, depending on what was done. No special reimbursement is provided if radiofrequency is used. Codes vary with lesion size, benign or malignant characteristics, location, and type of removal. Some lesions would be billed out as true "excision." Others would be billed as "shave excision," and still others would be termed "destruction" or "biopsy." The reader is advised to consult the most recent CPT coding manuals and other sections of this text.

Chapter 10

Ingrown Nail Removal

COMMON INDICATIONS

A wedge excision of the margins of the great toe nail is performed to treat recurrent infection of the ingrown nail. Ablation of the outer edges of the nail matrix with electrocautery or chemical cautery can prevent recurrence of an ingrown nail. The anatomy and terminology of the nail are detailed in Figure 10-1.

FIGURE 10-1. Anatomy.

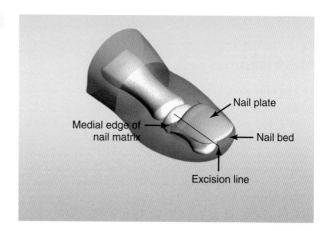

EQUIPMENT

Iris scissors, suture scissors, a hemostat, and a local anesthetic tray are needed for this procedure. Straight iris scissors are preferred, but curved scissors can also be used (Figure 10-2).

FIGURE 10-2. Equipment.

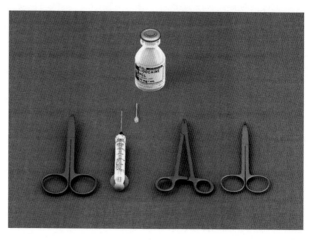

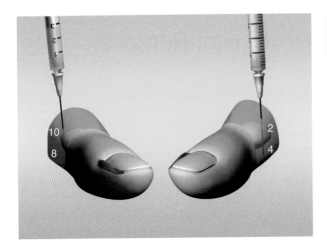

FIGURE 10-3. Dual nerve block in a single pass on each side of toe (through 2 o'clock and 10 o'clock positions)

KEY STEPS

1. **Preparation:** Cleanse the toe with an antiseptic solution.

2. **Anesthesia:** Perform a digital block of the great toe by passing the needle ventrally alongside the base of the proximal phalanx of the great toe at 2 o'clock and 10 o'clock positions. Inject 2 to 3 cc on each side of the toe, passing the needle deep toward the 4 o'clock and 8 o'clock positions, respectively (Figure 10-3). Take care to avoid direct intra-arterial injection of anesthetic by aspirating before injection. Inject 2 to 3 cc along the needle track while pulling the needle back toward the skin surface. This will block all four digital nerve branches.

3. **Lifting edge of ingrown nail:** Slide a single blade of the iris scissors between the nail bed and the nail plate along the ingrown area (Figure 10-4). A perceptible strain occurs when the tip of the scissors has passed the proximal edge of the nail. When this occurs, use a pair of straight mosquito hemostats to grasp the nail. With firm pressure holding the nail plate to the nail bed, the affected edge is carefully rolled out to extract the ingrown portion of the nail out of its compartment (Figure 10-5).

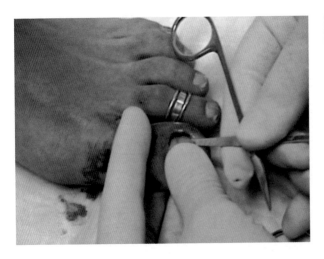

FIGURE 10-4. Lift nail edge using iris scissors.

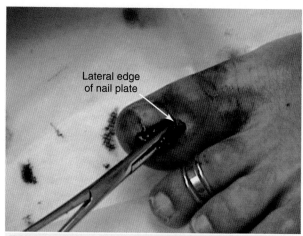

Lateral edge
of nail plate

FIGURE 10-5. Roll out lateral nail edge with a hemostat.

4. **Removal of ingrown nail edge:** Use suture scissors to trim the uplifted nail plate edge back to the base of the nail plate (Figure 10-6). Ensure that the entire portion of the nail segment to be removed has been excised down to the nail matrix.

5. **Ablation of the matrix:** Phenol ablation is the most common method used to cauterize the nail matrix to prevent or retard future growth of the unwanted portion of the nail. A small plug of cotton can be formed by trimming the cotton from the tip of swab and soaking it with phenol. The plug is inserted into the opening left by the excised nail edge and pushed into the germinal matrix to cauterize the area (Figure 10-7). When the matrix is cauterized, the cotton plug must be removed.

6. **Dressing:** Cover the toe with a padded bandage, and instruct the patient to soak daily in warm water and wear open-toe shoes for several days until the toe no longer feels tender.

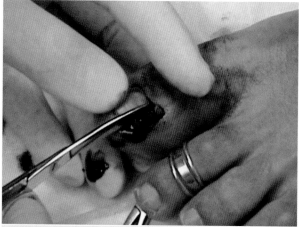

FIGURE 10-6. With heavy scissors, cut nail back to the matrix.

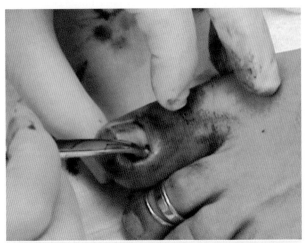

FIGURE 10-7. Ablation of matrix with a phenol-soaked cotton plug.

ICD-9 CODES

703.0   Nails, Ingrown

Obstetrics

Chapter 11

Vaginal Delivery

COMMON INDICATIONS

A vaginal delivery begins with the second stage of labor, which begins when the cervix is fully dilated. Confirm that the cervix is fully dilated by performing a cervical examination. During the second stage, uterine contractions and maternal pushing efforts move the fetus down from the pelvis to the introitus (Figure 11-1). The patient can begin pushing or is allowed to labor down for a period of time. The patient has several positions that she can use during the second stage. She can push in the squatting, supported supine, or side position.

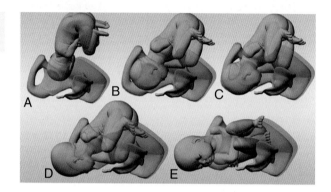

FIGURE 11-1. A-E. Cardinal movement of the fetus during the second stage of labor.

EQUIPMENT

The key equipment needed for a routine vaginal delivery includes a bulb suction, gauze, two hemostats for cord clamping, scissors for cutting the cord, and ring forceps to extract membranes or to aid in the examination after delivery. Instruments for suturing a laceration should also be included in the delivery kit (Figure 11-2). While the patient is pushing, prepare your equipment for delivery. Make preparations for the active management of the third stage of labor and immediate newborn care after delivery. Prepare the administration of pitocin for either 10 mg IM, 5 mg IV, or 20 mg IV in a liter of normal saline over 1 to 2 hours.

FIGURE 11-2. Equipment.

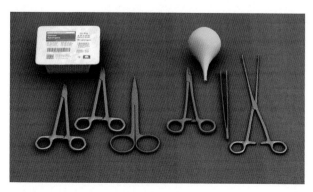

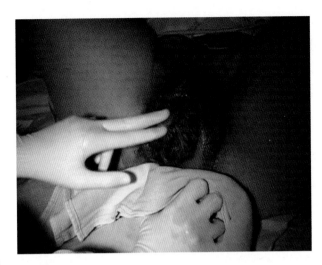

FIGURE 11-3. Controlled delivery of the head.

KEY STEPS

1. **Preparation:** The patient can lie on her back during the delivery, squat, or use stirrups, depending on her comfort with the position and the clinical situation. The squat position does not allow the physician to intervene easily, so it should be reserved for low-risk deliveries only.

2. **Anesthesia:** The patient may elect for no anesthesia, epidural, pudendal, or local blocks.

3. **Delivery of head:** As the infant's head begins to crown, use one hand to apply light pressure to the head. Control the delivery of the head with minimal contact, and do not resist the maternal forces that are pushing out the infant (Figure 11-3). There is no evidence that suggests supporting the perineum reduces the incidence of perineal lacerations.

4. **Delivery of anterior shoulder and remainder of infant:** As the head delivers, determine the natural position of the head with respect to the shoulders. Allow the head to rotate to a neutral position, and check for a nuchal cord. Grasp the head, and apply gentle downward and outward traction to deliver the anterior shoulder (Figure 11-4). As soon as the anterior shoulder appears below the pubis, lift the head and shoulders to deliver the posterior shoulder. Excessive downward traction can lead to brachial plexus injury or worsen a posterior laceration for the mother. Slide your most posterior hand under the trunk to support the delivery of the rest of the infant. Place the infant on the mother's abdomen if there are no concerns about the need for resuscitation. Dry the infant vigorously to stimulate respirations and to reduce heat loss.

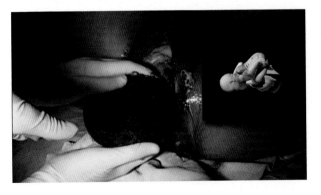

FIGURE 11-4. Delivery of the anterior shoulder.

FIGURE 11-5. Oxytocin administration (10 units IM).

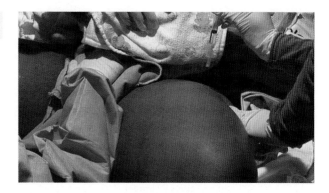

5. **Active management of the third stage (placental delivery):** Active management of the third stage includes three key steps:

   - Immediate pitocin administration
   - Controlled cord traction
   - Uterine massage after the placenta is delivered

   Delay cord clamping 2 to 3 minutes if the infant is stable. Clamp the umbilical cord in two places, and cut between the two clamps. Begin to apply controlled cord traction on the placental side of the cord as the uterus contracts. Check for any signs of hemorrhage or actively bleeding lacerations while waiting for the placenta to deliver. Use your left hand to apply pressure above the pubis against the uterine fundus. After separation, deliver the placenta, and slowly rotate the placenta and membranes to assist in extracting all of the membranes. Immediately begin the uterine massage to stimulate uterine contractions and further reduce the risk of hemorrhage (Figure 11-5).

6. **Immediate aftercare:** Inspect the cervix and perineum for lacerations (Figure 11-6). Every 5 minutes, check uterine tone and monitor maternal vital signs at gradually increasing intervals for the first 4 hours. Inspect the placenta for missing cotyledons, infarcts, or other abnormalities. Check to see that the membranes appear intact. The repair of lacerations and episiotomies is covered in Chapter 15.

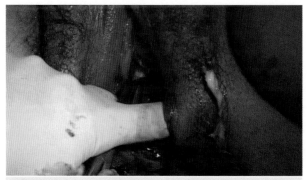

FIGURE 11-6. Inspection of the vagina for lacerations, using ring forceps.

ICD-9 CODES

Codes 630-677 cover "Complications of Pregnancy, Childbirth and Puerperium." Codes commonly used at the time of delivery have been selected below. The fifth digit is required for codes 640-676. For these codes, the following applies:

0 indicates unspecified as to episode of care.

1 indicates delivered with or without mention of antepartum condition.

2 indicates delivered, with mention of postpartum condition.

3 indicates antepartum condition or complication.

645.1	Postterm pregnancy (40-42 weeks)
645.2	Prolonged pregnancy (longer than 42 weeks)
649.1	Obesity complicating pregnancy, childbirth, or the puerperium
650	Normal delivery (not to be used with any other code in 630-676; fourth and fifth digits not required)
654.21	Previous cesarean section
656.31	Fetal distress
658.01	Oligohydramnios
659.21	Pyrexia in labor
662.01	Prolonged first stage of labor
662.21	Prolonged second stage of labor
663.01	Prolapse of cord
663.11	Cord around neck, with compression
664.11	Perineal laceration—second degree
664.21	Perineal laceration—third degree
664.31	Perineal laceration—fourth degree
666.12	Postpartum hemorrhage
667.12	Retained placenta/membranes
792.3	Meconium staining

Chapter 12

Amniotomy

COMMON INDICATIONS

Amniotomy is the artificial rupture of membranes performed in the course of labor. The most common reasons to perform an amniotomy are to assess amniotic fluid and to allow the placement of internal monitoring devices (Figure 12-1).

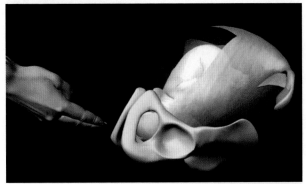

FIGURE 12-1. Amniotomy can be used to assess amniotic fluid.

EQUIPMENT

The amnio-hook is a plastic device that facilitates the artificial rupture of membranes (Figure 12-2).

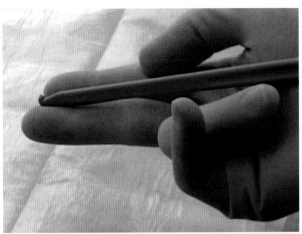

FIGURE 12-2. Amnio-hook.

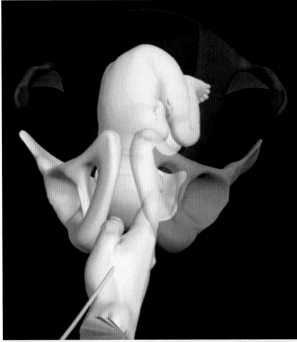

FIGURE 12-3. Cervical exam.

KEY STEPS

1. **Assess the cervix:** With sterile lubricated gloves, the cervix needs to be examined to assess the presenting part and cervical dilation (Figure 12-3). The cervix should be at least 2 cm dilated with the vertex well applied to the cervix.

2. **Confirm that fetal head is well applied:** An amniotomy should not be performed if the fetal head is not well applied to the cervix. Inappropriate amniotomy can increase the risk of a prolapsed cord.

3. **Insert vaginal fingers:** With the examining hand, identify the cervix and fetal vertex.

4. **Introduce amnio-hook:** With the other hand, pass the amnio-hook over the vaginal fingers, and snag the membranes with gentle traction (Figure 12-4). Leave the vaginal fingers in place while the amniotic fluid flows out.

5. **Prevent cord prolapse:** Confirm the absence of the prolapsed cord, and monitor the fetal heart rate for changes (Figure 12-5). Evaluate the amniotic fluid for meconium, and document the procedure.

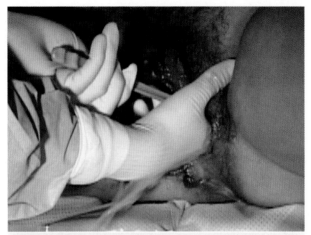

FIGURE 12-4. Snag the membranes with the amnio-hook.

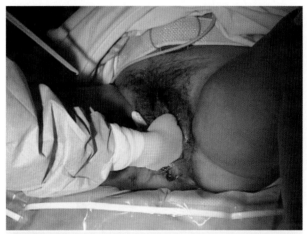

FIGURE 12-5. Leave fingers in place to detect a possible cord prolapse.

ICD-9 CODES

656.83   Meconium-stained fluid, affecting management of pregnancy or delivery, antepartum complication

656.83   Fetal distress, no other symptoms, affecting management of pregnancy or delivery, antepartum complication

657.03   Polyhydramnios, antepartum condition or complication

661.11   Secondary uterine inertia, arrested active phase of labor or hypotonic uterine dysfunction, delivered with or without mention of antepartum condition

662.01   Prolonged labor, first stage, delivered with or without mention of antepartum condition

662.21   Prolonged labor, second stage, delivered with or without mention of antepartum condition

Chapter 13

Scalp Lead Placement

COMMON INDICATION

Intrapartum fetal monitoring with continuous fetal heart rate monitoring can be occasionally difficult to obtain through the maternal abdomen. In these situations, a fetal scalp electrode can be placed to directly evaluate the fetal heart rate pattern.

EQUIPMENT

The bipolar fetal scalp electrode has a short spiral wire that can be twisted into the fetal scalp and then connected to a monitoring device (Figure 13-1).

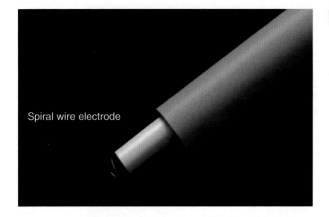

FIGURE 13-1. Equipment.

Spiral wire electrode

KEY STEPS

1. Open electrode kit: Carefully open the fetal scalp electrode container (Figure 13-2).

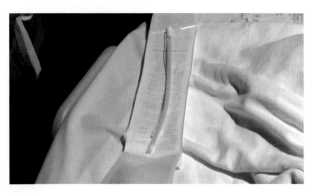

FIGURE 13-2. Open the electrode kit.

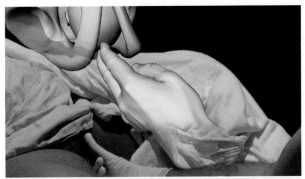

FIGURE 13-3. Cervical exam.

2. **Examine cervix:** To place a scalp electrode, the amniotic sac needs to be ruptured and the cervix sufficiently dilated to allow placement. With sterile gloves, gently place two lubricated fingers through the vagina and examine the fetal scalp. Confirm that the presenting part is the vertex (Figure 13-3).

3. **Place electrode on fetal scalp:** Place the tips of the index finger and middle finger directly on the fetal scalp. Be sure not to trap the vaginal skin and the cervix between the tips of the fingers and the fetal head. Supinate the vaginal hand, and slide the introducer containing the electrode over the palm. Carefully guide the introducer along the index finger and middle finger, and place the end of the introducer perpendicular to the fetal scalp. With the nonvaginal hand, turn the electrode 360° in a clockwise direction. The electrode will spin freely within the introducer (Figure 13-4).

4. **Withdraw introducer:** When the electrode is in place and anchored in the scalp, withdraw the introducer, being careful not to dislodge the electrode (Figure 13-5).

5. **Connect electrode:** After ensuring that the electrode is placed on the scalp, connect the electrode to the monitoring device (Figure 13-6).

6. **Electrode removal:** To remove the electrode, cut the wires with scissors, and separate the wires or twist them in a counterclockwise direction.

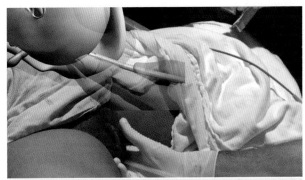

FIGURE 13-4. Place electrode on the fetal scalp.

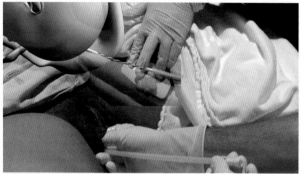

FIGURE 13-5. Withdraw the introducer.

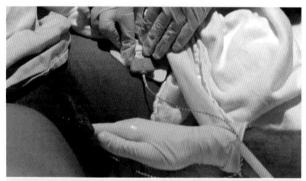

FIGURE 13-6. Connect the electrode to the monitoring device.

ICD-9 CODES

No ICD-9 codes are associated with this procedure.

Chapter 14

Intrauterine Pressure Catheter Placement

COMMON INDICATION

When it is not possible to fully assess the pressure of uterine contractions with external monitors, an intrauterine pressure catheter (IUPC) can be used. The IUPC provides a more accurate assessment of uterine contractions.

EQUIPMENT

The IUPC is packaged with the guide in a sterile kit (Figure 14-1).

KEY STEPS

1. **Cervical exam:** Explain the procedure to the patient, and gently examine the cervix. Confirm that the cervix is dilated at least 2 cm and that the membranes are ruptured. The artificial rupture of the membranes will be necessary if they are still intact. Set the baseline to "0." If amnioinfusion is planned, flush the amnioport with infusion solution (Figure 14-2).

2. **Place fingers on presenting part:** Pass the examining fingers through the introitus and cervix, and place the fingers against the fetal presenting part. If the location of the placenta is known, place the catheter on the opposite side of the uterus (Figure 14-3).

3. **Introduce the IUPC guide:** With the nonvaginal hand, insert the IUPC within the plastic guide along the palm of the vaginal hand through the introitus and cervix and cupped between the index finger and middle finger (Figure 14-4).

4. **Position the guide:** With the vaginal hand, gently advance the index finger and middle finger to place the plastic guide between the fingers and the presenting part. The nonvaginal hand should now gently thread the IUPC through the guide, past the presenting part and into the gestational sac. Stop advancing the IUPC when the 45-cm mark is at the introitus, or if resistance is noted (Figure 14-5).

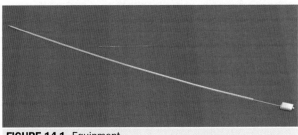

FIGURE 14-1. Equipment.

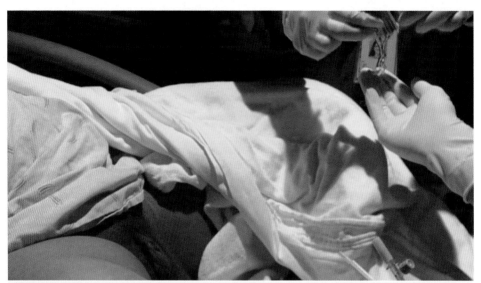

FIGURE 14-2. Cervical exam.

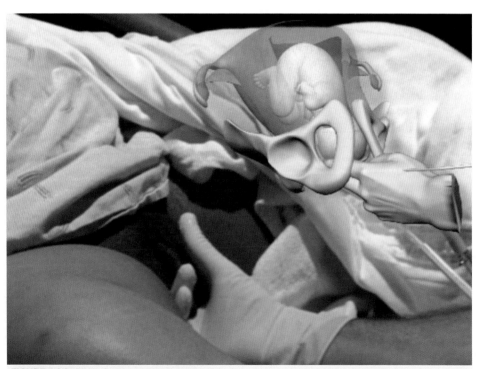

FIGURE 14-3. Place fingers on presenting part.

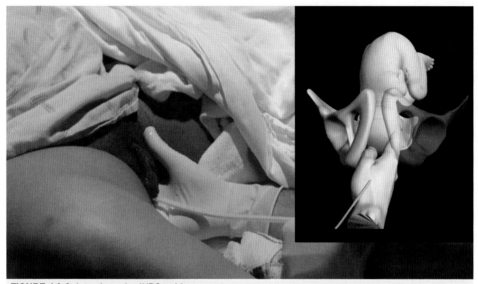

FIGURE 14-4. Introduce the IUPC guide.

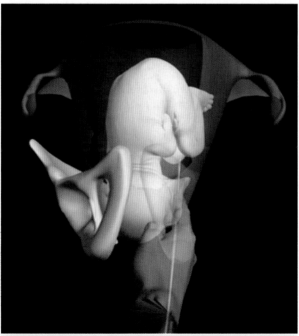

FIGURE 14-5. Position the guide and advance the catheter.

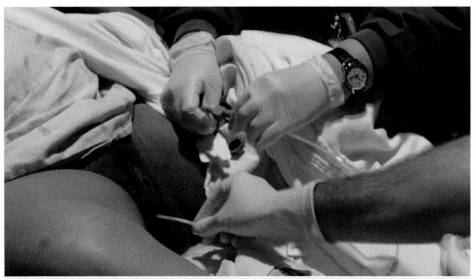

FIGURE 14-6. Remove the guide and connect the catheter to the monitor.

5. **Remove the guide:** When correctly positioned, use the nonvaginal hand to retract the catheter guide and remove it from the IUPC. Connect the IUPC to the monitor and secure the IUPC to the patient's thigh (Figure 14-6).

ICD-9 CODES

685.0X Oligohydramnios
658.4X Infection of amniotic cavity
661.0X Infection of amniotic cavity
662.1X Prolonged labor
665.1X Rupture of uterus during labor
792.3   Nonspecific abnormal findings in fluid surrounding fetus
        "X" indicates the need for a 5th digit for complete coding; 0, unspecified as to episode of care; 1, delivered; and 3, antepartum condition.

Chapter 15

First- and Second-Degree Laceration Repair

COMMON INDICATIONS

If an episiotomy is performed or a laceration occurs during delivery, a repair should be made to speed the recovery of the patient after delivery. Inspect the perineum to identify all lacerations and sources of bleeding. Control the bleeding before repairing the perineum. If the bleeding is coming from above the easily visualized area of the vagina, inspect the cervix to be sure that there are no cervical lacerations.

EQUIPMENT

The instruments required for a perineal repair include a needle driver and a tissue forceps such as a Russian forceps to grasp the needle while suturing (Figure 15-1). To prevent a needle stick injury, avoid using your fingers to grasp the needle during the entire repair. Use 3-O chromic gut or absorbable braided polymer suture such as Dexon or Vicryl for the repair. For deeper second-degree or greater lacerations, use absorbable braided polymers for the entire repair.

KEY STEPS

1. The vaginal apex, posterior fourchette (PF), and perineal apex are identified (Figure 15-2). It is critical that the two sides of the posterior fourchette are approximated during the repair. Consider performing a rectal exam with a double-gloved hand to confirm the thickness of the rectovaginal septum, then discard the outer glove. Inspect the full depth of the laceration or episiotomy to clearly identify the tissue layers and the degree of the laceration.

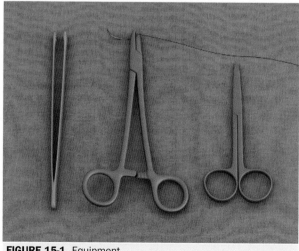

FIGURE 15-1. Equipment.

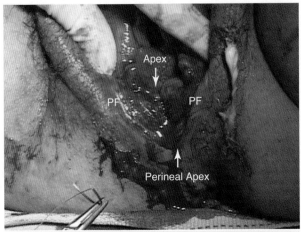

FIGURE 15-2. Identify the anatomy of the laceration.

2. A local anesthetic is injected along the edges of the laceration to provide a block for the repair. If an epidural is in place, a local anesthesia may not be required.

3. Place an anchoring stitch through the vaginal mucosa above the deep aspect of the laceration just above the apex of the tear or episiotomy (Figure 15-3). Use a continuous running suture to close the internal vaginal portion of the tear, working gradually outward toward the posterior fourchette (Figure 15-4). If the laceration is deep and approaches the anterior rectal wall, you may need to perform a deep-layer closure above the rectum in the rectovaginal septum. If this is done, be sure that all stitches are placed in the septal tissue and that none penetrate the rectal space.

4. When near the posterior fourchette, direct the suture deep toward the tissue anterior to the rectal sphincter to begin a deep-layer closure of the perineal aspect of the laceration. Run the stitches posteriorly in the subcutaneous and deep layers down to the posterior aspect of the tear. For this layer, insert the needle about 5 mm below the skin surface, drive it deep

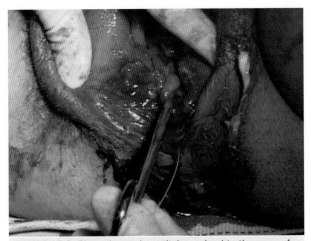

FIGURE 15-3. Place the anchor stitch proximal to the apex of the laceration.

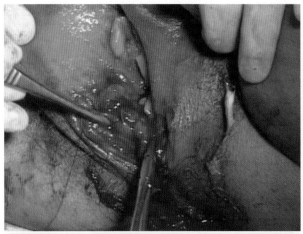

FIGURE 15-4. Completed vaginal wall repair.

along the same side about 1 cm, cross over deep on the opposite side, then bring the needle out at the 5-mm level on the opposite side from the start of the suture (Figure 15-5). Bring the needle entry posteriorly and across about 1 cm for the next suture.

5. When the deep-layer closure is completed, repair the perineal body using a subcuticular closure in the posterior to anterior direction along the perineal body. The suture is run continuously to the posterior fourchette until the skin is fully closed (Figure 15-6, A, B).

6. After the external skin is closed, the suture is brought up into the vaginal mucosa and anchored with another stitch along the posterior vaginal wall to bury the knot (Figure 15-7).

7. After the repair is completed, double glove one hand and perform a digital rectal exam to test the integrity of the repair and to ensure that no sutures were placed through the rectal mucosa. Dispose of the glove after the exam to ensure that you do not contaminate the patient (Figure 15-8).

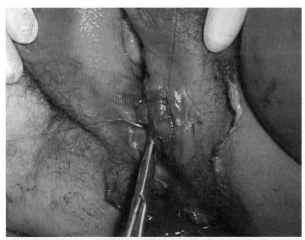

FIGURE 15-5. Deep closure of the laceration.

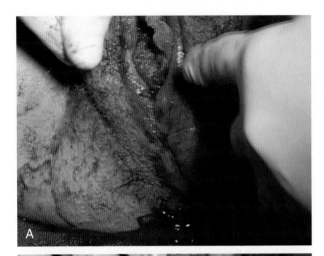

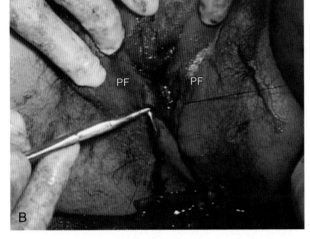

FIGURE 15-6. Repair of the (A) perineal body and (B) posterior fourchette.

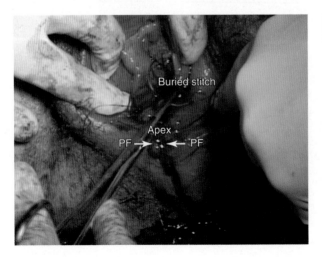

FIGURE 15-7. Bury the knot in the vagina.

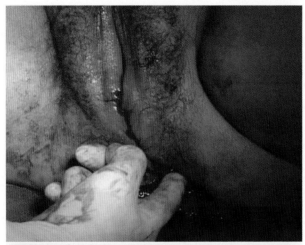

FIGURE 15-8. Perform a rectal exam after completion of the repair.

8. The patient is cleaned, and the amount of lochia is noted to ensure that bleeding is well controlled. Pain and swelling of the perineum should be controlled with oral analgesics and ice packs, as needed.

ICD-9 CODES

No ICD-9 codes are associated with this procedure.

Chapter 16

Vacuum-Assisted Delivery

COMMON INDICATIONS

Vacuum-assisted delivery is commonly indicated to assist in the completion of the second stage of labor for patients with an inadequate propulsive force to deliver their infants. The physician should clearly identify the indication for the procedure, which most often includes maternal exhaustion, fetal distress, or soft tissue dystocia that impairs the descent of the infant. The risks of the procedure—cephalohematoma, maternal lacerations, pelvic floor trauma, fetal intracerebral injury, and a failed attempt at instrumented delivery with the requirement of a cesarean delivery—should all be discussed with the mother as part of the consent for the procedure.

EQUIPMENT

There are several vacuum devices in use for vacuum-assisted delivery. They all include an application surface cup that attaches to the fetal head, a handle where traction is applied, and a suction mechanism, either inherent in the device or one connected to the device through tubing that is connected to the suction. For non-outlet vacuums, devices with a freely rotating cup allow for a higher station for application (Figure 16-1).

KEY STEPS

1. **Apply cup to flexion point:** Determine the fetal head position and station. The fetal head must be fully engaged in the pelvis and ideally at least +2 station. Place a pudendal block for anesthesia if no other block is present. Ensure that the cervix is fully dilated and that

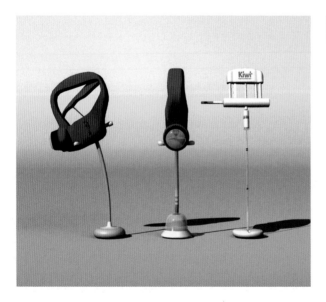

FIGURE 16-1. Common vacuum devices.

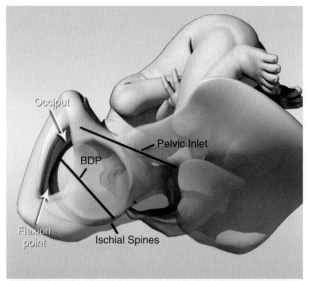

FIGURE 16-2. Flexion point in an occiput anterior delivery at +3 station.

the bladder is empty. Consider whether an episiotomy is indicated to expedite the delivery. Identify the presenting part of the fetal head and the fontanelle that is most easily palpated. The flexion point is located 3 cm anterior to the posterior fontanelle on the fetal head (Figure 16-2). This point must be identified because it is the ideal placement site for the vacuum cup. If the cup is applied to the flexion point, the head will often restitute properly when traction is applied, even in occiput posterior presentations (Figure 16-3, A-C). Note that the flexion point is often more posterior than commonly thought, so consider

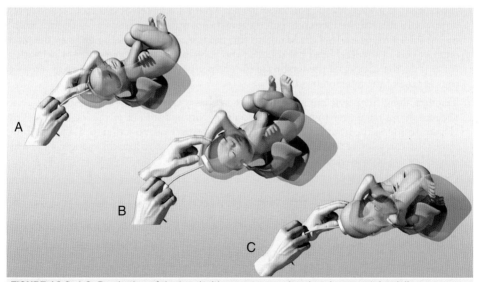

FIGURE 16-3. A-C. Restitution of the head with a vacuum-assisted occiput posterior delivery.

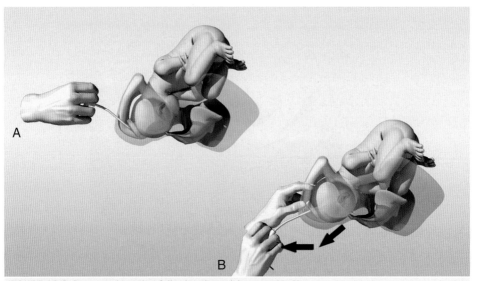

FIGURE 16-4. Downward traction following the pelvic curve (*A*, *B*).

this carefully when applying the cup. To apply the cup, use the first two fingers of the left hand to separate the labia. Use the right hand to insert the cup posteriorly along the vaginal wall, with the cup facing the fetal head. When over the flexion point, use the right hand to apply the cup to the scalp and activated suction to seal the cup on the fetal scalp. Check the margins of the cup to make sure that no vaginal sidewalls are entrapped before applying traction.

2. **Application of traction:** Apply your left thumb on the suction cup and index finger on the scalp to assist in maintaining the suction seal (Figure 16-4, A). Increase the suction to the range that is ideal for the particular device. Wait for a maternal contraction and apply downward and outward traction to pull the fetal head, with the assistance of maternal pushing, as shown in Figure 16-4, B. Maintain this traction angle with each pull until the most anterior part of the fetal head has rounded the pubic bone. In occiput anterior deliveries, this will be the occiput of the fetal head. In occiput posterior deliveries, this will often be the very top of the fetal forehead.

3. **Traction along the pelvic curve:** After the head has rounded the pubis, begin to raise the vacuum in a J maneuver to bring the presenting part upward out of the vaginal opening (Figure 16-5). As the head crowns, slowly control the pace of extraction to allow stretching if the fetus can tolerate the delay. When the head is delivered, reduce the suction, and break the seal of the vacuum device.

4. **Completion of delivery:** Continue by delivering the shoulders and the rest of the infant, as per a routine delivery (Figure 16-6). Anticipate shoulder dystocia in any patient who requires an instrumented delivery.

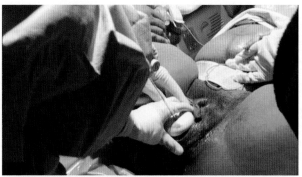

FIGURE 16-5. Completion of J maneuver with crowning of the head.

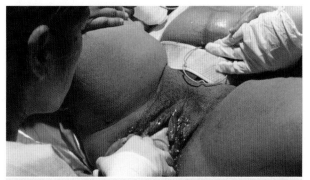

FIGURE 16-6. Delivery of the anterior shoulder.

ICD-9 CODES

669.51   Forceps or vacuum delivery

Chapter 17

Forceps Delivery

COMMON INDICATIONS

A forceps delivery is commonly indicated to assist in the completion of the second stage of labor for patients with inadequate propulsive force to deliver their infants. The physician should clearly identify the indication for the procedure, which most often includes maternal exhaustion, fetal distress, or soft-tissue dystocia that impairs the descent of the infant. The risks of the procedure—facial trauma for the infant, maternal lacerations, pelvic floor trauma, fetal intracerebral injury, and the failed attempt at instrumented delivery with the requirement of a cesarean delivery—should all be discussed with the mother as part of the consent for the procedure (Figure 17-1).

EQUIPMENT

Simpson's forceps are the most widely accepted outlet forceps in use. There are three parts to the forceps: handle, shanks, and blades. The two blades articulate just above the handles. Unpack the two blades from the sterile pack, and reconnect them to ensure that you have a complete set of forceps before proceeding (Figure 17-2).

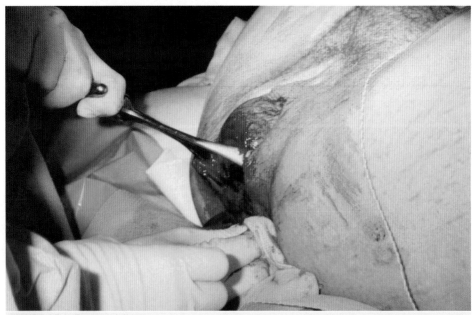

FIGURE 17-1. Forceps delivery.

FIGURE 17-2. Simpson's forceps (fenestrated).

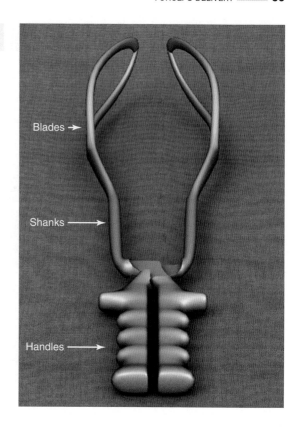

Blades →

Shanks ⟶

Handles ⟶

KEY STEPS

1. **Preparation:** Determine the fetal head position, station, and rotation, if present. Consider the use of a pudendal block for anesthesia, if no other block is present. Ensure that the cervix is fully dilated and that the bladder is empty. Anticipate that a shoulder dystocia could occur with any assisted delivery. Consider whether an episiotomy is indicated or whether it is likely needed to expedite the delivery. It is optimal to cut a mediolateral episiotomy to reduce the risk of rectal sphincter injury.

2. **Insertion of the left blade:** The left blade is first inserted, using the left hand to grasp the left blade handle, and the right hand is inserted into the vagina to protect the left maternal sidewall during insertion. Insert the blade flat on the posterior aspect of the vagina, and use the internal hand to guide the blade laterally and deep around the fetal head (Figure 17-3, A, B).

3. **Insertion of the right blade:** Repeat the same steps on the opposite side, with the right hand on the blade handle and the left hand protecting the sidewall (Figure 17-4).

4. **Prepare to apply traction:** Rearticulate the blades and ensure that they are aligned. Check that the blades are aligned with the sagittal suture and that there is only a finger tip of space between the blade and the fetal head. In occiput anterior presentations, the posterior fontanelle should be about 1 cm above the shanks of the blades (Figure 17-5).

5. **Forceps traction:** Apply downward and outward traction following the pelvic curve, also known as *Pajot's maneuver*. After the head has rounded the pubis, begin to raise the forceps handles in a J maneuver to bring the presenting part upward out of the vaginal opening.

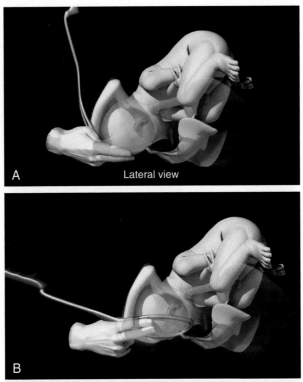

FIGURE 17-3. Maternal left blade insertion (*A, B*).

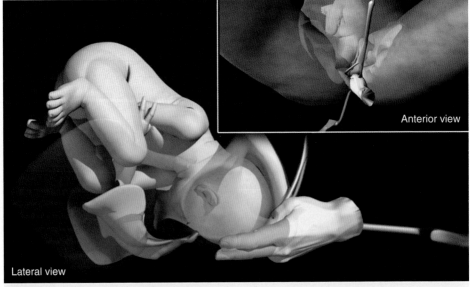

FIGURE 17-4. Right blade insertion.

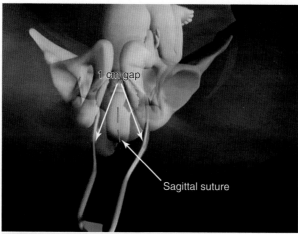

FIGURE 17-5. Alignment for traction application.

As the head crowns, slowly control the pace of extraction to allow stretching if the fetus can tolerate the delay. When the shanks are nearly vertical, check to see whether the jaw is delivered posteriorly, then disarticulate and remove the blades (Figure 17-6).

6. **Completion of delivery:** Continue by delivering the shoulders and the rest of the infant, as per a routine delivery.

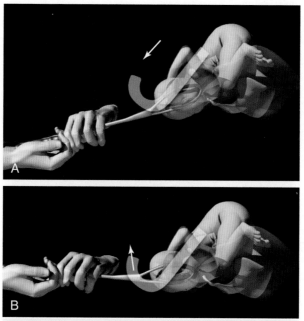

FIGURE 17-6. A-B. Traction with the J maneuver (Pajot's).

ICD-9 CODES

Codes 630-677 cover "Complications of Pregnancy, Childbirth and Puerperium." Codes commonly used at the time of delivery have been selected below. The fifth digit is required for codes 640-676. For these codes, the following applies:

0 indicates unspecified as to episode of care.
1 indicates delivered with or without mention of antepartum condition.
2 indicates delivered, with mention of postpartum condition.
3 indicates antepartum condition or complication.

645.1	Postterm pregnancy (40-42 weeks)
645.2	Prolonged pregnancy (longer than 42 weeks)
649.1	Obesity complicating pregnancy, childbirth, or the puerperium
650	Normal delivery (not to be used with any other code in 630-676; fourth and fifth digits not required)
654.21	Previous cesarean section
656.31	Fetal distress
658.01	Oligohydramnios
659.21	Pyrexia in labor
662.01	Prolonged first stage of labor
662.21	Prolonged second stage of labor
663.01	Prolapse of cord
663.11	Cord around neck, with compression
664.11	Perineal laceration—second degree
664.21	Perineal laceration—third degree
664.31	Perineal laceration—fourth degree
666.12	Postpartum hemorrhage
667.12	Retained placenta/membranes
792.3	Meconium staining

Chapter 18

Third- and Fourth-Degree Laceration Repair

COMMON INDICATIONS

Third- and fourth-degree perineal lacerations occur when the head of the infant applies excessive tension to the perineal body and the posterior fourchette during delivery. Episiotomies are rarely cut to the third degree, but the extension of second-degree episiotomies to third- or fourth-degree lacerations is relatively common. The third-degree laceration results in the tearing of the external and internal rectal sphincters, and the fourth-degree tear involves the rectal mucosa (Figure 18-1).

EQUIPMENT

A standard delivery set with a Russian forceps, needle driver, a Gelpi retractor, and Alice clamps is ideal for this repair. Plan to repair the rectal mucosa with 4-O or 5-O chromic gut. The rectal fascia should be repaired with 3-O Vicryl or Dexon to provide tensile strength for at least 2 weeks. Repair the rectal sphincter with 2-O Vicryl or Dexon (Figure 18-2). The remaining final closure of the second-degree repair is reviewed in Chapter 15, which covers vaginal laceration and episiotomy repair.

KEY STEPS

Fourth-Degree Repair

1. **Inspection:** Carefully inspect the laceration, and identify the rectal mucosa, the rectal submucosal fascia, and the internal rectal sphincter with its fibrous capsule. Grasp the torn

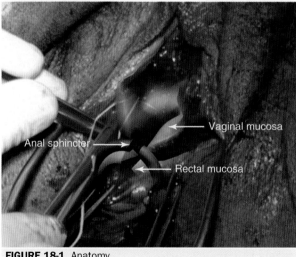

FIGURE 18-1. Anatomy.

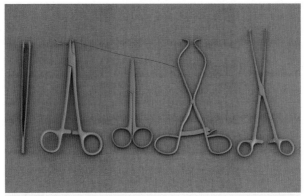

FIGURE 18-2. Instruments.

ends of the rectal sphincter with the Alice clamps to prevent them from retracting into the capsule. Use the Gelpi retractor to open the laceration above the rectal mucosa to allow for clear, hands-free visualization of the area to be repaired.

2. **Mucosal closure:** Begin suturing the rectal mucosa by anchoring a stitch proximally above the mucosa tear, using 4-O or 5-O chromic gut. Begin a running stitch through the mucosal layer, taking fine bites about 2 mm from the edge of the tear and 2 mm between each suture. Run the entire length of the tear, and continue the repair through the anal skin past the pectinate line (Figure 18-3).

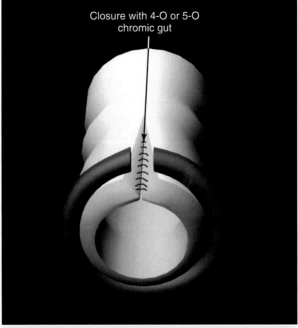

Closure with 4-O or 5-O chromic gut

FIGURE 18-3. Mucosal closure

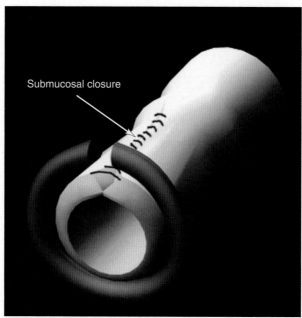

FIGURE 18-4. Submucosal closure

3. **Submucosal fascia closure:** Return to the proximal apex of the repair, and close the submucosal fascia layer of the rectum with 3-O braided synthetic suture with a similar running stitch. Take care not to pass the suture through the mucosal repair. This suture layer should be anterior to the mucosal closure in its entirety (Figure 18-4).

After completing these two layers, the closure now evolves into the third-degree repair.

Third-Degree Repair

The rectal sphincter and capsule are repaired together because the sphincter muscles alone are friable, and capsular tissue is needed to add strength to the repair.

1. **Inspection:** Begin the repair by pulling together the Alice clamps that are holding each side of the tear. Identify the superior aspect of the capsule on each side. A figure-of-eight stitch with 2-O braided synthetic suture will be done on three aspects of the sphincter to provide six points of tension across the sphincter closure (Figure 18-5).

2. **Sphincter repair:** Pass the needle through the superior aspect of the capsule on the patient's left, coming out through the sphincter muscle and crossing over to the opposite side. Pass the needle into the sphincter, then exit the capsule. Bring the suture back to the patient's left side, pass through the capsule then sphincter again, cross to the right side, and come through the sphincter and capsule again in the proper order (Figure 18-6). Securely tie the figure-of-eight stitch. This completes the posterior-superior knot. Repeat the same process for the inferior aspect of the capsule and sphincter. This secures the sphincter closest to the rectal mucosa, taking care not to pass the suture beyond the actual sphincter. Finally, place a figure-of-eight knot anteriorly over the sphincter and capsule, which will complete the third-degree closure (Figure 18-7).

The remaining final closure of the second-degree repair is reviewed in Chapter 15.

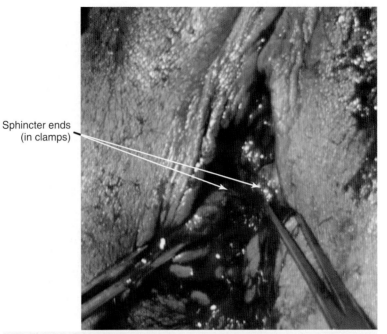

Sphincter ends
(in clamps)

FIGURE 18-5. Sphincters in clamps

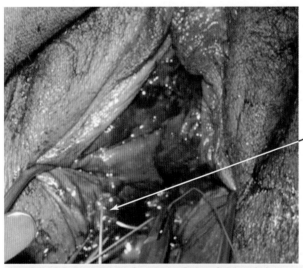

Completion of posterior
figure-of-eight stitch

FIGURE 18-6. Completion of posterior figure-of-eight stitch.

Completion of three figure-of-eight stitches

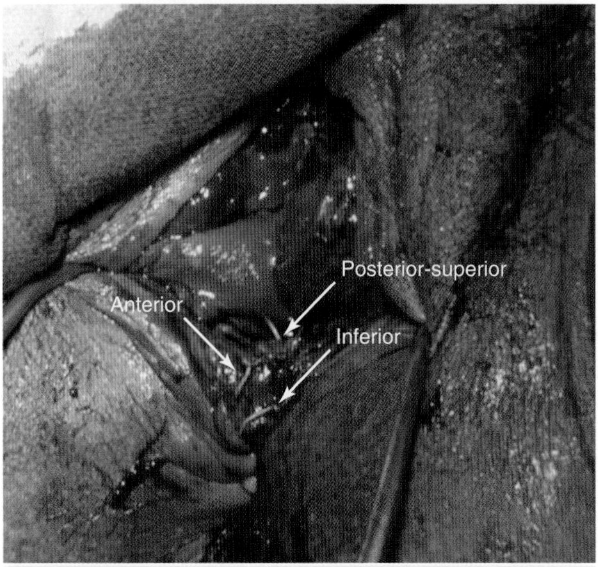

FIGURE 18-7. Final image of three figure-of-eight closures of the sphincter.

ICD-9 CODES

650 Normal delivery
The fifth digit (X) is required for Codes 660-669 to denote the following:

0 Unspecified
1 Delivered, with or without mention of antepartum condition
2 Delivered, with mention of postpartum complication
3 Antepartum condition or complication
4 Postpartum condition or complication

Codes related to delivery with forceps or vacuum:

662.2X Prolonged second stage of labor
659.7X Abnormality in fetal heart rate or rhythm

Codes related to episiotomy and episiotomy repair and to repair of low vaginal lacerations:

664.0X First-degree perineal laceration
664.1X Second-degree perineal laceration
664.2X Third-degree perineal laceration
664.3X Fourth-degree perineal laceration
664.4X Unspecified perineal laceration

Chapter 19

Cesarean Section

COMMON INDICATIONS

A cesarean section is required when labor fails to progress normally or when there is fetal distress. Other indications include eclampsia, severe preeclampsia, breech infants, and multiple gestations. The indications will impact the type of anesthesia used for the operative delivery. The patient should have epidural, spinal, and general anesthesia delivered by an anesthesiologist who is trained in obstetrical anesthesia.

EQUIPMENT

A complete abdominal surgical tray should be used for cesarean sections. Individual instrument preferences for specific steps of the procedure are common and should be noted in the surgeon's preference card. Use O-chromic suture for both layers of the uterine closure because the evidence best specifically supports this suture type.

KEY STEPS

1. **Preparation:** Place the patient in the supine position with a right lumbosacral lift to tilt the uterus off the inferior vena cava. Prepare the entire lower abdomen and inguinal areas, and drape the patient in a sterile manner. There is a wide variety of materials and drape sets that are available; familiarity with your site-specific drapes is important (Figure 19-1).

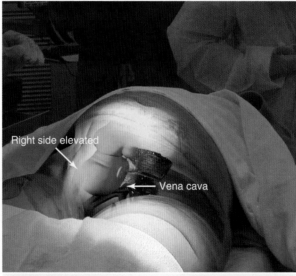

FIGURE 19-1. Preparation.

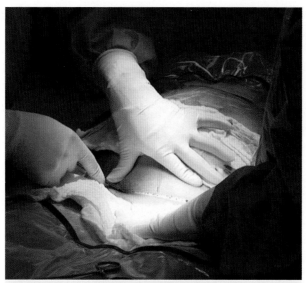

FIGURE 19-2. Skin incision 2 cm above the pubis.

2. **Skin and fascia incision:** Test the skin and ensure that the patient has complete anesthesia of the operative area. With a No. 10 blade scalpel, make a Pfannenstiel incision 2 cm above the pubic ramus, usually about 15 cm in length (Figure 19-2).

The incision size should be adjusted based on the patient's habitus and estimated fetal size. Incise the skin and subcutaneous fat down to the fascia. Expect to encounter the inferior epigastric arteries and veins along the lateral aspects of the incision line. These can be either clamped or cauterized for hemostasis. Open the fascia adjacent to the midline linea alba. Incise the fascia down to the rectus muscle, then use Metzenbaum or curved Mayo scissors to bluntly track laterally along the incision path, separating the fascia off the rectus muscle. The scissors are then used to extend the initial fascia incisions laterally, approximating 10 cm in each direction (Figure 19-3). The assistant should use a small

FIGURE 19-3. Fascia incision.

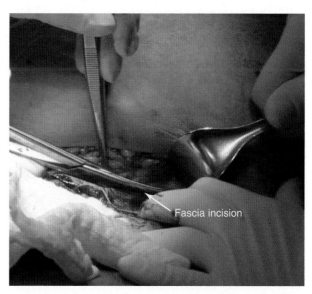

Fascia incision

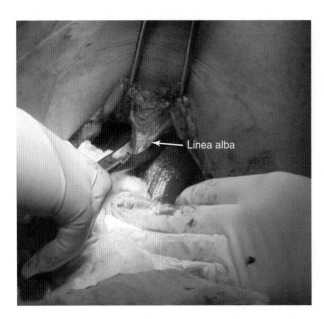

FIGURE 19-4. Releasing the linea alba.

Linea alba

retractor to provide lateral exposure for the surgeon to create an adequate fascia incision. When the fascia is opened, it is manually dissected superiorly and inferiorly off the rectus. The linea alba will remain attached at the midline. Clamp the fascia with Kocher clamps and lift the fascia off the rectus, providing counter-traction against the linea alba. Using heavy Mayo scissors, cut the linea alba free, both superiorly and inferiorly from the rectus muscle. Take care not to button-hole the fascia when releasing it from the linea alba (Figure 19-4).

3. **Entry into peritoneum:** Divide the midline of the rectus muscle and the pyramidalis muscle sharply along the vertical axis using scissors, and manually separate them to expose the peritoneum. Using pick-ups or forceps, lift the peritoneum up and visually confirm the absence of bowel below the thin peritoneal layer. Create a small opening with Metzenbaum scissors or bluntly with the fingers to enter the abdominal cavity (Figure 19-5). After opening the peritoneum, visualize the bladder inferiorly, and place the bladder blade to expose the lower uterine segment. Make a 15-cm transverse incision over the peritoneum that overlies the lower uterine segment. Manually separate the reflection

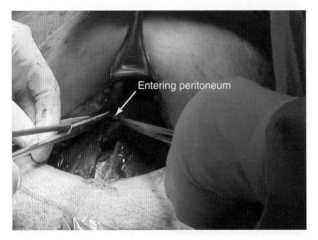

FIGURE 19-5. Entry into the peritoneum.

Entering peritoneum

FIGURE 19-6. Incision into visceral peritoneum overlying the uterus.

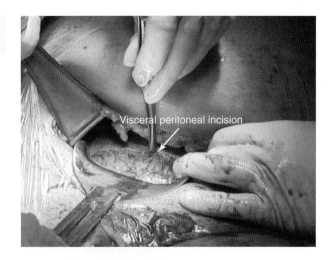

FIGURE 19-6. Incision into visceral peritoneum overlying the uterus.

of the peritoneum from the lower uterus to create the bladder flap. The bladder blade is replaced into the bladder flap to protect the bladder and provide exposure for the uterine incision (Figure 19-6).

4. **Uterine incision:** There are several methods to enter the uterus. In this case, the uterine incision is initially scored over the lower uterine segment, then the center of the incision is carefully expanded layer by layer until the myometrium is completely incised. Often the membranes will bulge up through the incision when the uterine cavity is entered. If the fetal head is closely applied to the lower segment, care must be taken to avoid lacerating the fetal scalp or face. When the uterine cavity is entered, place a finger in each side of the incision, and extend the incision laterally and upward, avoiding extension to the lateral margins of the uterus where the uterine arteries are located. The bladder blade is removed before the delivery of the infant (Figure 19-7).

5. **Delivery of infant and placenta:** Place a hand into the incision, and grasp the fetal presenting part. In a typical vertex presentation, grasp the fetal head. Bring the head to the uterine incision, and apply fundal pressure and direct traction on the flexed fetal head to deliver the

FIGURE 19-7. Uterine incision.

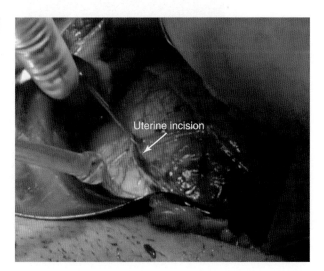

head through the uterine incision. Deliver the rest of the infant. Suction the oropharynx as soon as the infant's mouth is exposed to reduce the risk of aspiration of amniotic fluid. Clamp the cord in two places, and cut the cord between the clamps. While maintaining sterility, hand the infant to an attendant for management of its care. Obtain cord blood samples if needed. Deliver the placenta with gentle cord traction or by manual extraction. Using ring forceps, remove membranes that may be adherent to the endometrium. Use a dry lap sponge to sweep the uterine cavity for any clots or remaining membranes. The patient should receive 30 units of IV pitocin given at a rate of 10 units per hour after the placenta is delivered (Figure 19-8, A, B).

6. **Closure of the uterus:** Now that delivery is complete, close the uterus expeditiously. With ring forceps, grasp the corners of the uterine incision and the superior and inferior edges of the incision. Replace the bladder blade within the bladder flap to protect the bladder during closure. Close the uterus with O-chromic or synthetic polymer absorbable suture, using a locking stitch. Using O-chromic has a lower risk of uterus dehiscence in subsequent labor

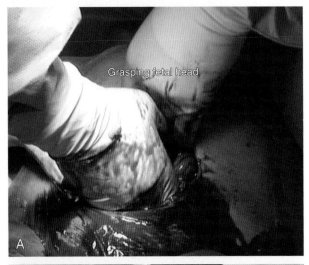

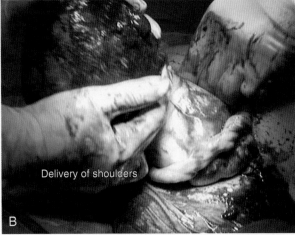

FIGURE 19-8. A-B. Delivery of an infant.

episodes. Place the first stitch at the lateral apex of the uterine incision on the patient's left. Avoid suturing through the uterine artery, which may be in close proximity to this lateral margin. Palpating and identifying the location of the uterine artery can help avoid accidental penetration of the artery when placing these sutures. Tie the suture with four knots to secure the anchor stitch. Tag the anchor stitch for easier access later in the closure. Using a locking stitch, run the suture transversely across the uterus, taking full thickness bites through the myometrium during the closure (Figure 19-9, A). After the first layer is completed, create an imbricating layer to reinforce the closure. Imbrication can be done with a horizontal imbricating stitch or a vertical imbricating stitch. A vertical imbricating stitch can be performed in a single pass by passing the needle into the myometrium above and below the first layer closure, if a large enough suture needle has been selected as shown in the inset. Continue to run the imbricating stitch transversely across the uterus, burying the first closure layer. After the uterus is closed, inspect the wound for bleeding and, if present, place figure-of-eight sutures around the sites to gain hemostasis (Figure 19-9, B).

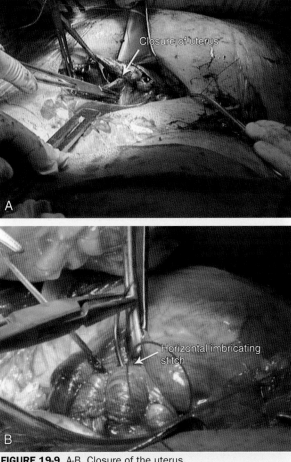

FIGURE 19-9. A-B. Closure of the uterus.

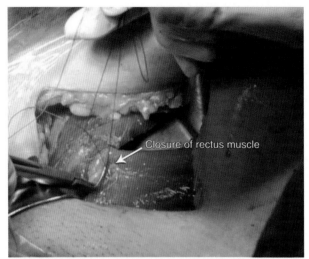

FIGURE 19-10. Closure of the rectus with a single 3-0 Dexon figure-of-eight stitch.

7. **Closure of peritoneum:** Inspect the uterus, fallopian tubes, ovaries, and the appendix at this time, and remove any blood from the peritoneal cavity. Inspect the pelvic gutters for accumulation of fluid or blood during delivery. Irrigate the gutters to remove blood, which can act as an irritant. If you choose to close the peritoneum, place two 3-O running chromic stitches to close this layer. Close the lower rectus muscle with two 3-O interrupted chromic stitches to reduce the risk of diastasis of the rectus muscles (Figure 19-10).

8. **Closure of the fascia and skin:** Close the fascia using O-Vicryl or similar synthetic polymer absorbable suture in a nonlocking running stitch. Ensure that the apices of the incision are fully visualized during closure and that they are closed completely. The assistant should use a small retractor to provide such exposure. Next close the subcutaneous layer with 3-O synthetic polymer absorbable suture. This reduces the risk of seroma formation in patients with more than 2 cm of adipose tissue overlying the lower abdomen. Finally, close the skin with either staples or a running subcuticular stitch. The running subcuticular closure is cosmetically appealing but requires more time to perform such a closure (Figure 19-11, A, B).

9. **Postoperative care:** All patients should receive intraoperative antibiotic prophylaxis with a second generation cephalosporin such as Cefazolin. If allergic to cephalosporins, use clindamycin and an aminoglycoside. After the surgery is completed, dress the wound and massage the fundus to express blood or clot from the uterus before the patient is sent to recovery. The patient may begin to eat after 8 to 12 hours and advance her diet as tolerated. Encourage ambulation the following day.

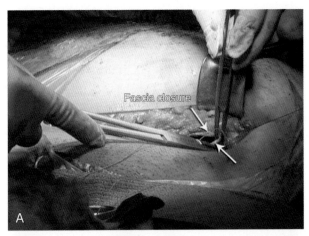

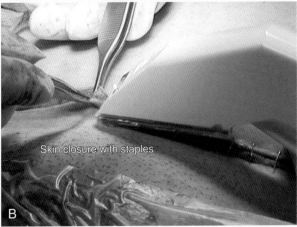

FIGURE 19-11. A. Fascia closure with O-Vicryl. B. Skin closure.

ICD-9 CODES

74	Cesarean section and removal of fetus
	Code also any synchronous:
Hysterectomy	(68.3-68.4, 68.6, 68.8)
Myomectomy	(68.29)
Sterilization	(66.31-66.39, 66.63)
74.0	Classical cesarean section
74.1	Low cervical cesarean section
74.4	Cesarean section of other specified type

Women's Health

Chapter 20

Pap Smear

COMMON INDICATION

The Pap smear is a useful tool in screening for early signs and risk factors of cervical malignancy.

KEY STEPS

1. **Inspect introitus:** Using the Pap light, carefully inspect the external genitalia for any abnormality or lesions (Figure 20-1).

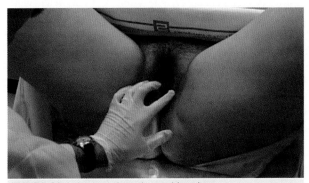

FIGURE 20-1. Inspect the vulva and introitus.

2. **Insert speculum:** Help the patient relax, and gently insert the speculum, moving it slowly to allow visualization of the cervix. If excess mucus is noted on the cervix, gently remove it with a cotton-tipped applicator to improve the accuracy of the test (Figure 20-2).

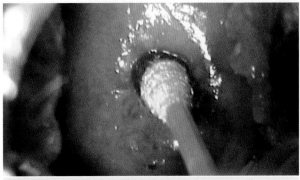

FIGURE 20-2. Remove excess mucus.

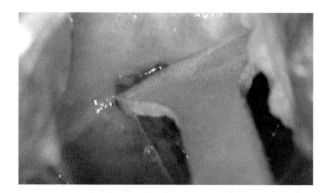

FIGURE 20-3. Rotate wooden spatula tip in the external os.

3. **Obtain sample:** Before obtaining the cell sample, label the frosted end of the glass slide with the patient's identifying information, such as name and date of birth. Using a wooden or plastic spatula, gently place the tip of the spatula against the cervical os, and rotate it 360° to collect a sample of cells (Figure 20-3). The sample is then spread evenly over a glass slide (Figure 20-4). Spray the slide immediately with fixative (Figure 20-5). Do not allow the glass slide to dry before applying the fixative. Air drying will cause the cells to enlarge and make interpretation difficult or impossible.

4. **Endocervical brush:** A cervical brush can be used to obtain endocervical cell samples. Gently place the brush tip in the endocervical canal, and rotate it 360° (Figure 20-6). Roll the brush onto a glass slide, and immediately spray it with a fixative.

5. **Human papillomavirus (HPV) sampling:** Use a broom-shaped applicator, and gently rotate it several times across the cervix (Figure 20-7). After smearing one side of the brush on a glass slide, place the tip of the brush inside the wet prep container labeled with the patient's name. Send samples to the cytology laboratory and for HPV typing, as indicated. If a visual abnormality is noted on the cervical inspection, the Pap smear may not serve as an adequate screening test, and the patient should be examined by colposcopy.

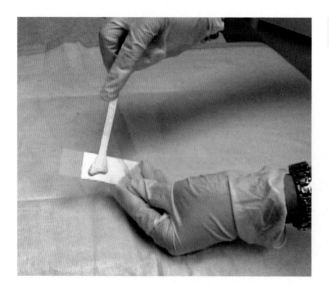

FIGURE 20-4. Spread cells on the labeled glass slide.

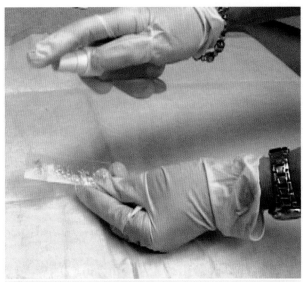

FIGURE 20-5. Spray fixative.

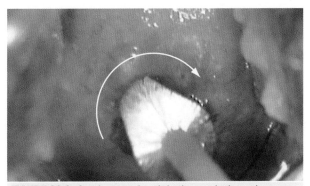

FIGURE 20-6. Gently rotate brush in the cervical canal.

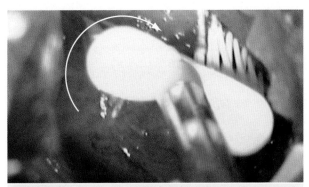

FIGURE 20-7. Gently rotate HPV broom on the cervix.

ICD-9 CODES

622.0	Cervical ulcer
622.10	Cervical dysplasia, unspecified
622.11	Mild dysplasia of cervix
622.12	Moderate dysplasia of cervix
622.2	Cervical leukoplakia
622.7	Cervical polyp
622.8	Cervical atrophy
623.8	Abnormal vaginal bleeding
626.8	Uterine bleeding
233.1	Cervical carcinoma in situ, severe dysplasia of cervix
795.0	Abnormal Pap (some insurances will not reimburse for this code)
219.0	Neoplasm of the cervix, benign
180.9	Malignant neoplasm of the cervix, unspecified
V15.89	Other specified personal history presenting hazards to health; other (for high-risk patients)
V76.2	Special screening for malignant neoplasms; cervix
V76.47	Special screening for malignant neoplasms; vagina

Chapter 21

Vulvar Biopsy

COMMON INDICATIONS

Vulvar lesions that are not identifiable as benign or that fail to respond to therapy should be biopsied for a definitive diagnosis and treatment (Figure 21-1).

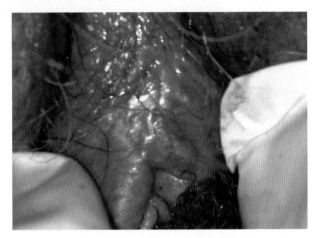

FIGURE 21-1. Biopsy vulvar lesions for a definitive diagnosis.

KEY STEPS

Punch biopsy instrument, small Adson's forceps or pick-ups, small iris scissors, and a specimen jar can be used to sample these lesions. Lidocaine solution of 1%, with or without epinephrine, a syringe, and a 25-gauge needle will be necessary for anesthesia. Monsel's solution and cotton-tipped applicators are usually sufficient for hemostasis (Figure 21-2).

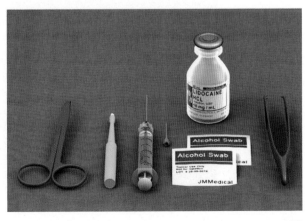

FIGURE 21-2. Equipment.

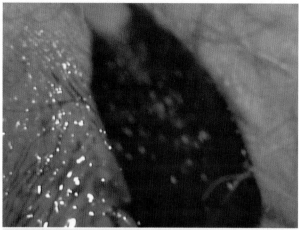

FIGURE 21-3. Cleanse lesion.

KEY STEPS

1. **Anesthetize the lesion:** If the patient is not allergic to iodine, clean the lesion with Betadine (Figure 21-3). Slowly inject 1 to 2 cc of lidocaine under the lesion, elevating it slightly (Figure 21-4).

2. **Perform punch biopsy:** Select a suitable-sized punch biopsy instrument to obtain a sufficient sample for a diagnosis such as 3 or 4 mm. Gently rotate the punch through the dermal layer to the subcutaneous fat (Figure 21-5). Use the small Adson's forceps or pick-ups to gently lift the sample core and excise it with small iris scissors (Figure 21-6). Place the sample in a labeled specimen jar, and inspect the punch biopsy site (Figure 21-7).

3. **Wound care:** Hemostasis can usually be achieved with pressure or with the application of Monsel's solution (Figure 21-8). Submit the sample for a pathologic evaluation.

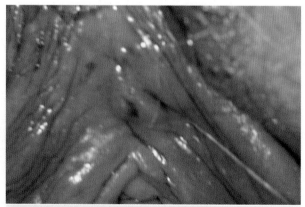

FIGURE 21-4. Inject lidocaine analgesia.

FIGURE 21-5. Rotate punch biopsy to obtain a sample of the lesion.

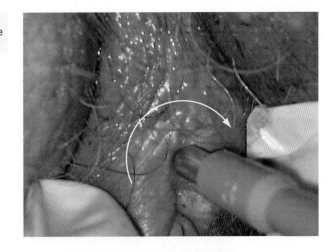

FIGURE 21-6. Excise sample with iris scissors.

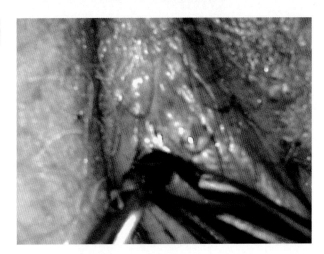

FIGURE 21-7. Punch biopsy site.

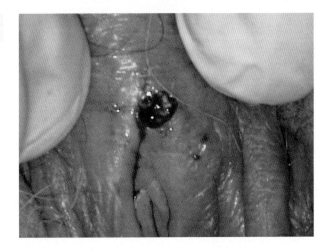

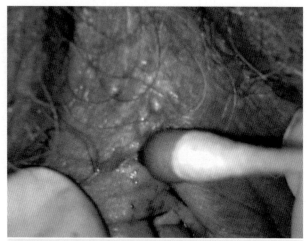

FIGURE 21-8. Apply pressure to stop superficial bleeding.

ICD-9 CODES

624.9	Unspecified noninflammatory disorder of vulva and perineum
078.11	Condyloma acuminatum
701.9	Skin tag
221.2	Benign vulvar neoplasm
624.01	Vulvar intraepithelial neoplasia I (VIN I)
624.02	VIN II
233.32	VIN III
616.10	Vulvitis

Chapter 22

Word Catheter Placement

COMMON INDICATIONS

Bartholin's cyst abscesses can be treated by two methods. Word catheter placement is the first-line therapy for an infected Bartholin's gland. If infections recur or if Word catheter placement is not curative, then marsupialization of the gland is the most definitive therapy (Figure 22-1).

EQUIPMENT

The equipment required for the Word catheter placement includes a No. 11 or No. 15 blade scalpel, a hemostat, 5 cc of sterile water, a Word catheter, and 10 cc of a lidocaine and bupivacaine local anesthetic in a 1:1 mixture (Figure 22-2).

KEY STEPS

1. **Preparation and anesthesia:** Place the patient in the lithotomy position, and cleanse the perineum with antiseptic solution. Palpate the cyst to clearly visualize its size and location. Place a block over a 2-cm diameter area over the vaginal sidewall that overlies the surface of the cyst. If local cellulitis and induration are present, a small field block may provide optimal anesthesia (Figure 22-3).

2. **Incision:** Incise the vaginal sidewall with a 3-mm incision, using the scalpel blade through the mucosal layers and into the cyst. Remove the blade and use a small hemostat to enter the cyst, and hold the incision open to allow the contents to drain (Figure 22-4).

FIGURE 22-1. Anatomy.

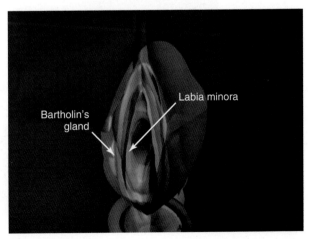

Labia minora

Bartholin's gland

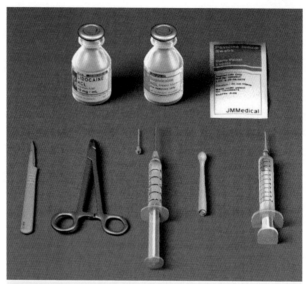

FIGURE 22-2. Equipment.

3. **Inflation of Word catheter:** Test the Word catheter balloon by filling the catheter with 3 cc of sterile water then allowing the syringe to refill and collapse the Word catheter balloon. With the balloon deflated and the catheter attached to the syringe, insert the tip of the catheter into the cyst cavity. Holding the incision open with the hemostat can aid in proper placement of the catheter. It is possible to place the catheter between the mucosal layer and the cyst if the insertion is not done correctly, which will not properly drain the cyst. Inflate the balloon with 3 cc of sterile water, and remove the needle from the base of the catheter. The catheter should stay in place, comfortably filling the cyst space. Be sure not to overfill the balloon and create high tissue tension around the cyst because it can cause significant patient discomfort after the anesthetic wears off (Figures 22-5 and 22-6).

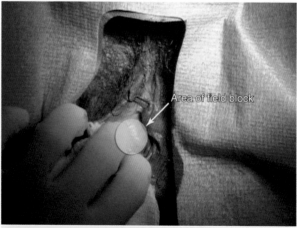

FIGURE 22-3. Area of anesthesia.

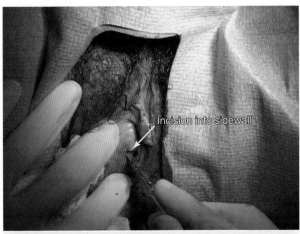

FIGURE 22-4. Incision into the cyst.

4. **Post-procedure care:** Push the catheter back into the vagina, and provide the patient with clear postoperative care instructions to ensure proper healing of the tract created by the Word catheter. The catheter is removed ideally at 3 weeks by simply deflating the balloon and removing the catheter (Figure 22-7).

5. **Dressing:** The patient should wear a perineal pad for several days while the catheter is draining.

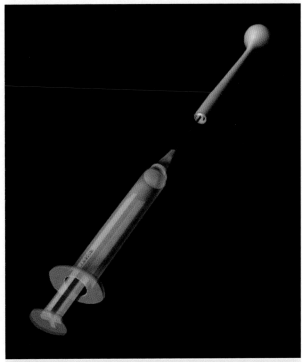

FIGURE 22-5. Test inflation of the catheter.

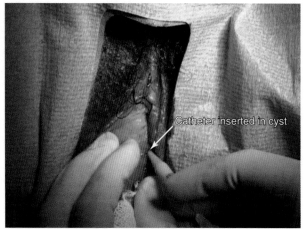

FIGURE 22-6. Insertion of the catheter.

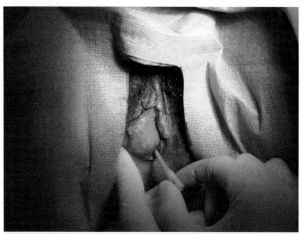

FIGURE 22-7. Post-procedure appearance.

ICD-9 CODES

616.2   Bartholin's cyst
616.3   Bartholin's abscess
616.4   Other vulvar abscess

Chapter 23

Bartholin's Marsupialization

COMMON INDICATIONS

Marsupialization of the Bartholin's gland is commonly performed for recurrent infections of the gland or failure of a Word catheter to adequately treat the problem. Word catheter placement is the first-line therapy for an infected Bartholin's gland. If infections recur or if Word catheter placement is not curative, then marsupialization of the gland is the most definitive therapy. Marsupialization can be done in the clinic setting or in same day surgery, depending on the patient's preference for anesthesia (Figure 23-1).

EQUIPMENT

The equipment required for marsupialization includes 10 cc of a lidocaine and bupivacaine local anesthetic 1:1 mixture with a long 27-gauge needle for injection, a minor surgery tray with a No. 15 blade scalpel, and 3-O absorbable braided suture such as Vicryl or Dexon (Figure 23-2).

KEY STEPS

1. **Preparation and anesthesia:** Place the patient in the lithotomy position, and cleanse the perineum with antiseptic solution. Palpate the cyst to clearly visualize its size and location. Place a block over a 2-cm diameter area on the vaginal sidewall that overlies the surface of the cyst. If local cellulitis and induration are present, a field block may provide optimal anesthesia.

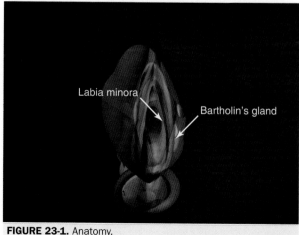

Labia minora

Bartholin's gland

FIGURE 23-1. Anatomy.

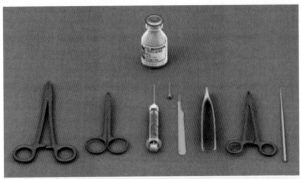

FIGURE 23-2. Equipment.

2. **Incision:** Outline the incision using a surgical marker just deep to the junction of the vaginal sidewall and labia minora. The incision should be a 2- to 3-cm ellipse whose long axis follows the internal axis of the vaginal sidewall, not involving the external labial skin. Use the No. 15 blade scalpel to create the elliptical incision. The vaginal mucosa is entered, followed by a careful incision through the fascia overlying the cyst. There are several layers of fascia and vaginal wall smooth muscles that will be divided in this process. These layers are opened sharply until the cyst wall is entered and begins to drain. When the cyst is entered and drained, the ellipse of tissue is fully excised, effectively removing the roof of the cyst that has been adjacent to the vaginal sidewall. What remains is the smooth cyst cavity with its distinct edge that must be clearly identified before closure begins (Figure 23-3A, B).

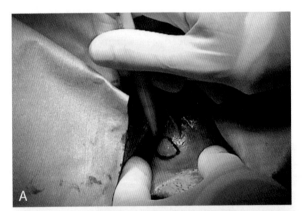

FIGURE 23-3. A-B. Marking and creating the incision over the cyst.

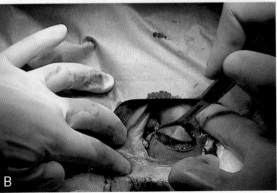

FIGURE 23-4. Identify the cyst wall and vaginal mucosa layers.

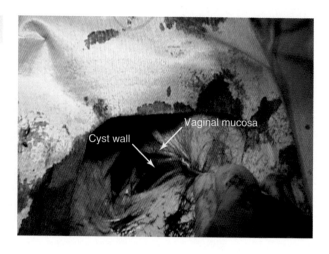

3. **Marsupialization:** Use 3-O Dexon or Vicryl to marsupialize the cyst. The initial stitch is placed by passing the needle though the mucosa and then passing through the cyst wall from the submucosal side to open the remaining portion of the cyst. The suture is run continuously around the margin of the incision in small 2- to 3-mm bites. The vaginal mucosa and cyst wall must be taken together in each stitch to properly marsupialize the tissue (Figures 23-4 and 23-5).

4. **Completion of suturing:** Continue to run the stitch around the full circumference of the ellipse. When the last stitch is placed, overlapping the initial anchoring stitch, the suture is securely tied off. At the completion of the procedure, note that the cyst wall is clearly opened and retracted by the circumferential stitches (Figure 23-6).

5. **Postoperative care:** Immediately postoperative, the appearance is that of a small cleft on the side where the surgery was performed (Figure 23-7). After several days, the repair is barely noticeable as the vaginal wall contracts further. The patient should perform daily sitz baths in warm water to keep the wound clean and follow up in 1 week for a postoperative check to ensure that the incision is healing well. Within 6 months, the wound will contract further and will appear as a nearly imperceptible opening on the vaginal sidewall.

FIGURE 23-5. Suturing the mucosa and cyst wall edge.

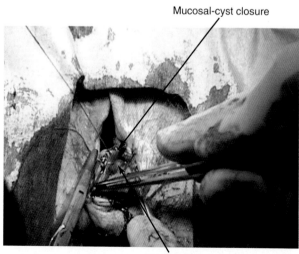

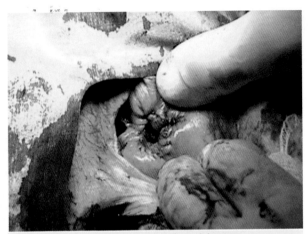

FIGURE 23-6. Completion of circumferential suture.

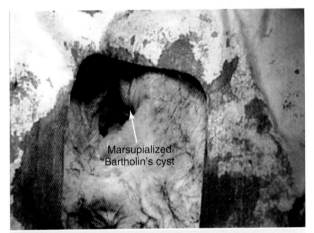

Marsupialized
Bartholin's cyst

FIGURE 23-7. Postoperative appearance.

ICD-9 CODES

616.2   Bartholin's cyst
616.3   Bartholin's abscess
616.4   Other vulvar abscess

Chapter 24

Cervical Polypectomy

COMMON INDICATIONS

Cervical polyps are usually benign pedunculated growths of the cervix that are often asymptomatic but can cause bleeding. Because they are occasionally malignant, small polyps are best removed during a gynecologic examination and sent to the pathology laboratory for diagnosis (Figure 24-1).

EQUIPMENT

Equipment includes a vaginal speculum, nonsterile gloves, ring forceps, a pathology container, and silver nitrate. Topical anesthesia is rarely necessary (Figure 24-2).

KEY STEPS

1. **Speculum:** Gently insert the vaginal speculum (Figure 24-3).
2. **Evaluate the polyp base:** Inspect the polyp with a cotton-tipped applicator or ring forceps to identify the base (Figure 24-4).
3. **Grasp with ring forceps:** If the polyp is cervical, gently grasp it with the ring forceps, and twist the forceps until the polyp is removed, and place it in the pathology container (Figure 24-5). Endometrial and large cervical polyps are best removed in a surgical suite or during a hysteroscopy.
4. **Control bleeding:** Bleeding can be controlled with direct pressure, Monsel's solution, or a silver nitrate application (Figure 24-6). The patient should be instructed to avoid intercourse and tampon use for 1 week and to return for reevaluation in 6 to 8 weeks.

FIGURE 24-1. Cervical polyp.

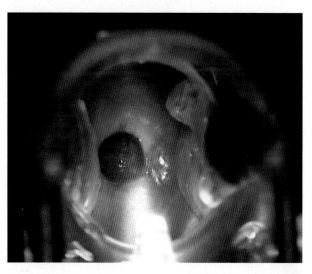

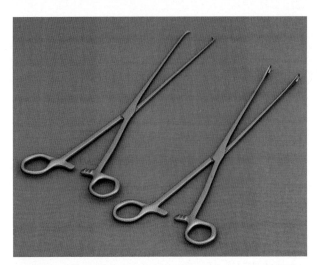

FIGURE 24-2. Ring forceps and tenaculum.

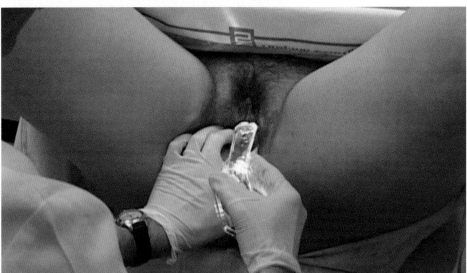

FIGURE 24-3. Gently insert the speculum.

FIGURE 24-4. Inspect the polyp with a cotton-tipped applicator.

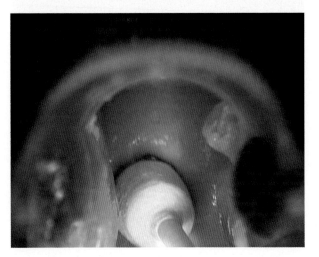

FIGURE 24-5. With ring forceps, gently grasp and twist the polyp at the base.

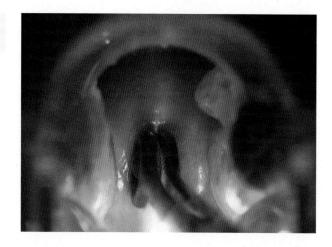

FIGURE 24-6. Control bleeding with direct pressure, Monsel's solution, or silver nitrate.

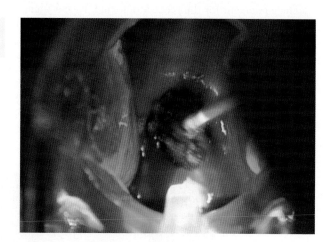

ICD-9 CODES

No ICD-9 codes are associated with this procedure.

Chapter 25

Endometrial Biopsy

COMMON INDICATIONS

An endometrial biopsy performed with a Pipelle catheter is an efficient way to sample the endometrium of the uterus with minimal discomfort to the patient (Figure 25-1). The most common reasons for performing an endometrial biopsy are to assess dysfunctional uterine bleeding and postmenopausal bleeding. Ensure that the patient is not pregnant before performing this procedure.

EQUIPMENT

The equipment for the procedure includes a speculum, a uterine sound, and a Pipelle catheter. A tenaculum may be necessary if the cervix is stenotic and countertraction is needed (Figure 25-2).

KEY STEPS

1. **Preparation:** Place the patient in the lithotomy position. Perform a bimanual exam to determine the orientation and size of the uterus. Insert a speculum, and visualize the cervix. Cleanse the cervix with antiseptic solution (Figure 25-3).

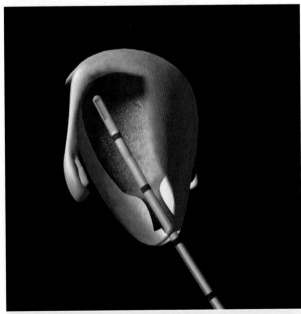

FIGURE 25-1. Pipelle catheter in the uterus.

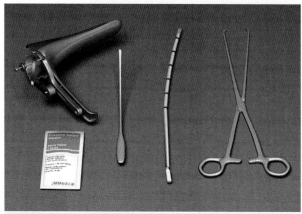

FIGURE 25-2. Equipment.

2. **Catheter insertion:** Use the uterine sound to dilate the os in most patients. You may first attempt to insert the Pipelle catheter if the os does not appear stenotic. Avoid contaminating the catheter on the vaginal sidewalls. Insert the catheter into the os to the fundus of the uterus. Countertraction using a tenaculum that is placed across the anterior lip of the cervix may be necessary if the os is firmly closed. The Pipelle catheter can be used as a sound to measure the depth of the uterus (Figure 25-4).

3. **Biopsy of the endometrium:** With the catheter inserted to the full depth of the uterus, pull back the plunger to create suction. Quickly advance and retract the catheter within the endometrial cavity while rotating the catheter between the fingers to obtain a full circumferential sample from all aspects of the endometrium. The bloody endometrial tissue should be drawn up into the catheter with this movement. Do not retract the catheter too far out of the uterus. If so, the negative pressure within the catheter will be lost. If this occurs early in the process, expel the contents of the catheter into a formalin container without contacting the formalin, then reinsert the catheter for another series of passes to collect an adequate sample (Figure 25-5).

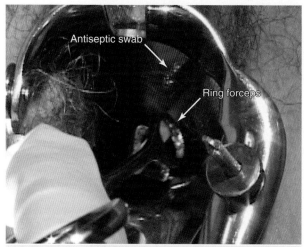

FIGURE 25-3. Preparation.

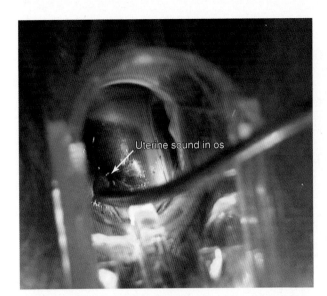

FIGURE 25-4. Dilating the os with a uterine sound.

Uterine sound in os

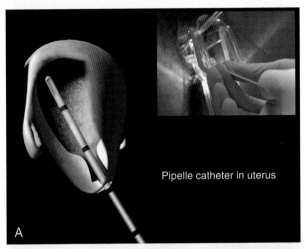

FIGURE 25-5. A. Insertion of the Pipelle catheter and application of suction. B. Contents of the uterus drawn into the catheter.

Pipelle catheter in uterus

A

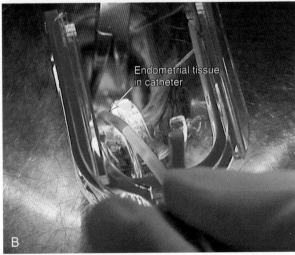

Endometrial tissue in catheter

B

FIGURE 25-6. Specimen is ejected into formalin.

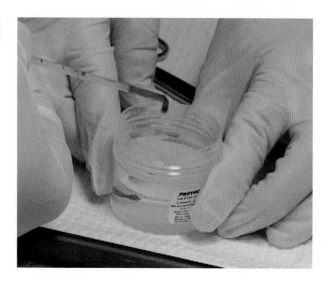

4. **Specimen collection:** When at least half of the catheter is filled with the endometrial sample, remove the catheter, and extrude the contents of the catheter into a formalin container for evaluation (Figure 25-6).

ICD-9 CODES

182.0	Insertion of cervical dilator (e.g., laminaria)
219.9	Benign neoplasm of uterus
233.2	Carcinoma in situ, uterus
236.3	Neoplasm of uncertain behavior, uterus
621.0	Polyp of endometrium
621.2	Hypertrophy of uterus; bulky or enlarged uterus
621.30	Endometrial hyperplasia, unspecified
620.31	Simple endometrial hyperplasia without atypia
621.32	Complex hyperplasia without atypia
621.33	Endometrial hyperplasia with atypia
625	Pain associated with female genital organs (requires a fourth digit and must be as specific as possible)
625.9	Unspecified symptoms associated with female genital organs
626.5	Ovulation bleeding; regular intermenstrual bleeding
626.6	Metrorrhagia; bleeding unrelated to menstrual cycle; irregular intermenstrual bleeding
626.8	Dysfunctional uterine bleeding
626.9	Unspecified uterine bleeding
627.0	Premenopausal menorrhagia
627.1	Postmenopausal bleeding
622.1	Atypical glandular cells
V07.4	Postmenopausal HRT
V10.41	Personal history of cancer of cervix, cancer of the uterus or endometrial cancer
VV10.40	Personal history of cancer of female genital organ, unspecified

Chapter 26

Intrauterine Device (IUD) Insertion

COMMON INDICATIONS

Intrauterine devices (IUDs) are an ideal option for women who desire a long-term, reliable solution for contraception. The primary use is in multiparous women who are done with childbearing, but many women who are nulliparous are now choosing IUDs for long-term (5 years or more) contraception. Ensure that the patient is not pregnant before performing this procedure (Figure 26-1).

EQUIPMENT

There are two common types of IUDs: copper T and Mirena. The Mirena IUD contains levonorgestrel as an adjunct to the mechanical effects of the IUD. The insertion techniques for these IUDs are similar with a few subtle design-related differences. The copper T arms must be flexed and folded into its insertion catheter. The Mirena IUD is pulled back into the insertion sheath, and the strings are locked at the base of the handle at the start of the procedure (Figure 26-2).

KEY STEPS

1. **Preparation:** Prepare the IUD for insertion in a sterile manner (Figure 26-3). Place the patient in the lithotomy position. Perform a bimanual exam to determine the orientation and size of the uterus. Insert a speculum and visualize the cervix. Cleanse the cervix with an antiseptic solution.

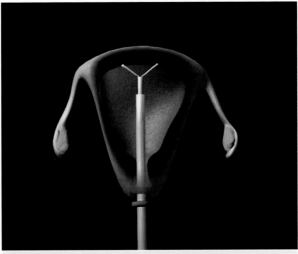

FIGURE 26-1. IUD during placement in the uterus.

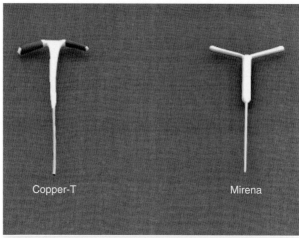

FIGURE 26-2. Types of IUDs (seen without applicators).

2. **Sounding of uterus:** Use the uterine sound to gradually dilate the os. Apply gentle pressure until the internal os relaxes. A palpable give is felt when this occurs. A tenaculum may be required for countertraction if the os is firmly closed. Always apply the tenaculum horizontally across the anterior lip of the cervix when it is used. Determine the depth of the top of the fundus with the sound. The marker ring on the IUD insertion catheter is set to match the sound results for both IUD types (Figure 26-4).

3. **Mirena IUD insertion:** When inserting the Mirena IUD, advance the IUD into the os until it is 1 cm short of the marker ring. Release the IUD strings from the base of the handle, and slide the blue advancement knob forward on the handle until it is 1 cm short of the top of the slide. Now, fully advance the IUD catheter to the marker, then push the IUD out of the catheter by fully advancing the blue knob on the handle forward up the

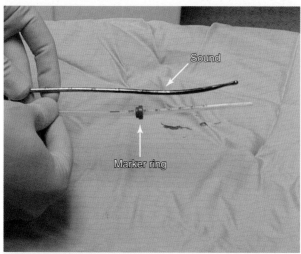

FIGURE 26-3. Preparation of the sound and IUD for insertion.

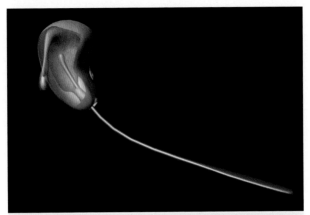

FIGURE 26-4. Uterine sound used to dilate os for IUD insertion.

slide (Figure 26-5). Be sure that the IUD strings are not locked or caught at the base of the handle before removing the insertion catheter. Remove the catheter and visualize the strings coming through the os. Trim the strings to 2 to 3 cm in length.

4. **Copper T IUD insertion:** When inserting the copper T IUD, advance the IUD until the ring is flush to the cervix. With the marker ring applied to the cervix, the center plunger is held still while the insertion catheter is withdrawn back over the plunger, expelling the IUD out of the insertion catheter (Figure 26-6). As the catheter is withdrawn fully, the strings should be visible coming through the os. Trim the strings to 2 to 3 cm in length.

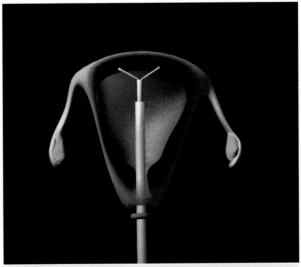

FIGURE 26-5. Mirena IUD at expulsion from the obturator.

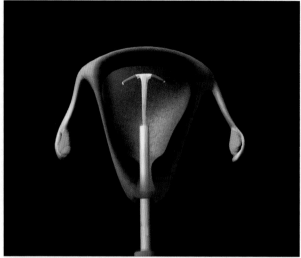

FIGURE 26-6. Copper T IUD after expulsion from the obturator.

ICD-9 CODES

V25.1 Insertion of intrauterine contraceptive device

Chapter 27

Intrauterine Device (IUD) Removal

COMMON INDICATIONS

Intrauterine devices (IUDs) are removed when they expire or if the patient develops unwanted side effects or complications. In most patients, the strings will still be visible and can be removed easily. Occasionally, the IUD strings are retracted up into the uterus and can no longer be used to remove the IUD. A more complex procedure is required.

EQUIPMENT

A ring forceps is used for a simple removal of the IUD with visible strings. The equipment needed for removing an IUD without visible strings includes a Cytobrush, local anesthetic, a 10-cc syringe, an 18- and 27-gauge needle with a needle extender, a uterine sound, a tenaculum, and an IUD hook (Figure 27-1).

KEY STEPS

1. **Removal of IUD with visible strings:** To remove an IUD with visible strings, first visualize the cervix with a speculum examination. Use a ring forceps to grasp the IUD strings, lock the forceps, then pull gently to remove the IUD from the uterus (Figure 27-2).

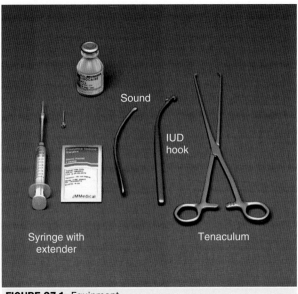

FIGURE 27-1. Equipment.

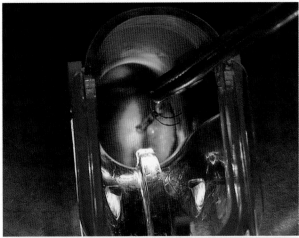

FIGURE 27-2. Removal with ring forceps when strings are visible.

2. **Removal of IUD without visible strings:**
   - First, perform a pelvic exam to ensure that the uterine position is known. Insert a vaginal speculum and visualize the cervix. Sweep the endocervical canal to see whether the strings can be retrieved. If not, cleanse the cervix with an antiseptic solution.
   - Place a two-quadrant or four-quadrant paracervical block, as shown in the paracervical block tutorial (Figure 27-3).
   - Using the uterine sound, determine the depth and internal shape of the uterus. The sound also dilates the os to allow the passing of the IUD hook (Figure 27-4).
   - Use an ultrasound image, if available, to find the location of the IUD with respect to the IUD hook. Identify the uterus and the IUD within the endometrial cavity (Figure 27-5).

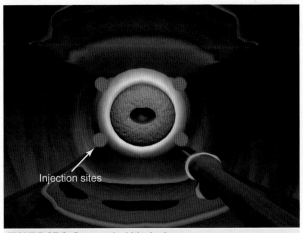

Injection sites

FIGURE 27-3. Paracervical block sites.

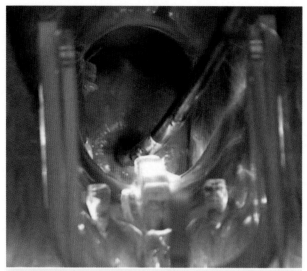

FIGURE 27-4. Sounding of the uterus.

- Insert the IUD hook to the top of the fundus. Attempt to feel for the IUD with the IUD hook in the fundus of the uterus. Pull the IUD hook out gently to see whether the strings or the IUD itself is caught within the hook. Several attempts will often be required. Again, the use of an ultrasound study can assist in determining whether the hook is anterior or posterior to the IUD, and guide and use pressure on the IUD hook to grasp the IUD. When the hook snags the IUD, carefully pull the IUD out through the os (Figure 27-6).

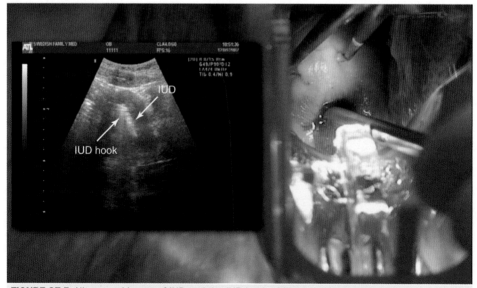

FIGURE 27-5. Ultrasound image of IUD and the IUD hook within the endometrial cavity.

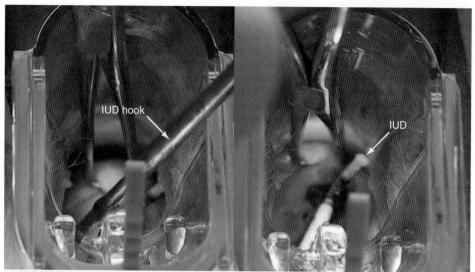

FIGURE 27-6. Extraction of IUD with a hook.

- The patient should be placed on prophylactic antibiotics with clindamycin or doxycycline for 3 days after the procedure to reduce the risk of infection.

ICD-9 CODES

V25.42 Intrauterine contraceptive (IUC) device; checking, reinsertion, or removal of intrauterine device (IUD)

Chapter 28

Breast Cyst Aspiration

COMMON INDICATIONS

Cystic breast nodules can be initially worked up and treated with aspiration. Persistent or recurrent nodules require further evaluation to rule out malignancy (Figure 28-1).

KEY STEPS

1. **Palpate the cyst:** Carefully and gently palpate the breast nodule.
2. **Prepare the skin:** Fully cleanse the skin with povidone-iodine or alcohol. Skin markers can be used to facilitate finding smaller cysts after the skin has been prepared (Figure 28-2).
3. **Stabilize the cyst:** Gently but firmly secure the cyst between the fingers of the nondominant hand (Figure 28-3).
4. **Topical anesthesia:** Anesthetize the skin's entry point with 1 to 2 cc of 1% lidocaine, with or without epinephrine, and inject down to the cyst wall.
5. **Aspirate the cyst:** Insert the needle into the center of the cyst, and withdraw the plunger to create a vacuum (Figure 28-4). After all of the cyst fluid is removed, apply direct pressure to the needle insertion site to prevent the formation of a hematoma (Figure 28-5). Send the sample to the cytology laboratory for evaluation. If any residual nodule is palpated, further workup should be arranged to rule out coexisting malignancy.

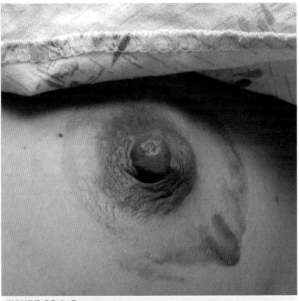

FIGURE 28-1. Breast cyst.

FIGURE 28-2. Prepare skin with povidone.

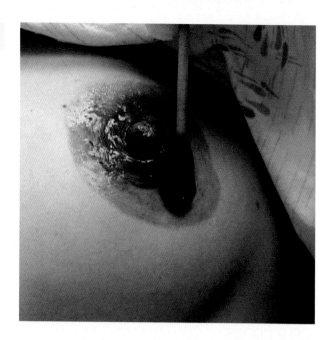

FIGURE 28-3. Stabilize the cyst with fingers.

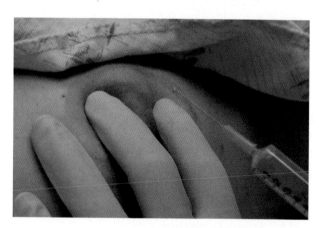

FIGURE 28-4. Aspirate the cyst.

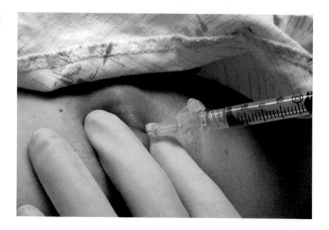

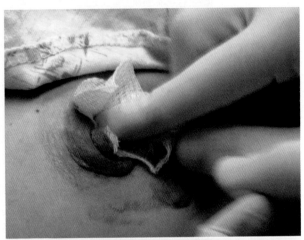

FIGURE 28-5. Apply direct pressure to site.

ICD-9 CODES

217	Benign lesion breast
610.0	Solitary cyst of breast
610.1	Fibrocystic breast disease
610.2	Fibroadenosis of breast
611.72	Breast lump
174.0	Cancer breast areola
174.1	Cancer breast central
174.2	Cancer breast upper inner quadrant
174.3	Cancer breast lower inner quadrant
174.4	Cancer breast upper outer quadrant
174.5	Cancer breast lower outer quadrant
174.6	Cancer breast axillary tail
193	Malignant neoplasm of thyroid
226	Benign neoplasm of thyroid
785.6	Enlarged lymph node

Chapter 29

Colposcopy Examination

COMMON INDICATIONS

Colposcopy is used to evaluate cervical abnormalities found on Pap smear cytology, visual screening with acetic acid, or to evaluate visible abnormalities (Figure 29-1).

EQUIPMENT

The instruments needed for this procedure include an adjustable vaginal speculum, an endocervical speculum, an endocervical curette, biopsy forceps, and small and large cotton-tipped swabs. A binocular colposcope provides optimal visualization and should have a green light filter. Use Monsel's solution for chemical cautery after biopsy (Figure 29-2).

KEY STEPS

1. **Preparation:** Place the patient in the lithotomy position, and insert a lubricated speculum. Clearly visualize the cervix, and focus the colposcope. Note any obvious abnormalities, and identify the transformation zone, the os, and the squamocolumnar junction (Figure 29-3).

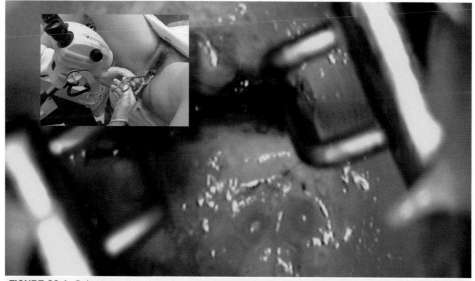

FIGURE 29-1. Colposcopy.

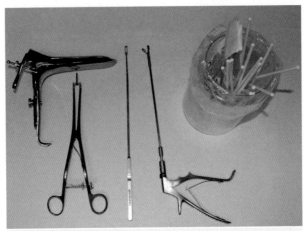

FIGURE 29-2. Equipment.

2. **Acetic acid application:** Apply 5% acetic acid to the cervix with two large swabs. Acetic acid converts potentially dysplastic epithelium to a whitish color within about 30 seconds. The cervix is then carefully inspected to look for any distinctive changes consistent with dysplasia. Acetowhite changes may take longer to develop in areas of high-grade dysplasia. Identify areas of fine mosaicism, coarse mosaicism, or punctuation. Green light examination allows for better visualization of a cervical vascular pattern (Figure 29-4A, B).

3. **Endocervical examination:** Examine the endocervical canal using an endocervical speculum to open the distal endocervical canal. The glandular endocervical epithelium can become faintly white; however, dysplasia appears more plaque-like and distinctly more acetowhite. Identifying lesions that lie within or extend into the endocervical canal is a critical requirement for a satisfactory colposcopy examination (Figure 29-5).

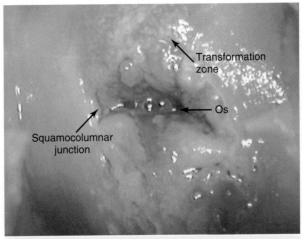

FIGURE 29-3. Anatomy of the cervix.

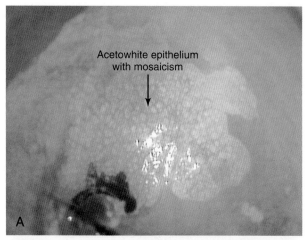

Acetowhite epithelium
with mosaicism

A

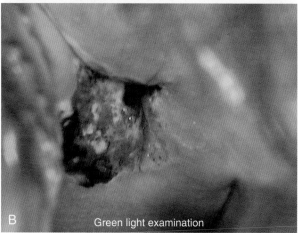

B

Green light examination

FIGURE 29-4. A. Acetowhite epithelium with mosaicism.
B. Green light examination.

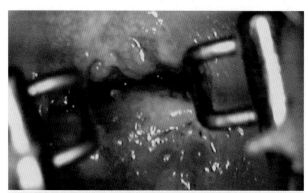

FIGURE 29-5. Endocervical examination.

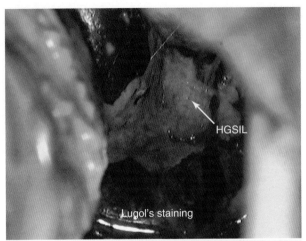

FIGURE 29-6. Lugol's staining with high-grade squamous intraepithelial lesion.

4. **Lugol's application:** Concentrated Lugol's iodine solution is also a useful adjunct in highlighting abnormal areas in patients without iodine allergy. Saturate swab, then paint entire surface. Dry cervix lightly after staining to remove residual Lugol's solution. Areas that stain dark brown are normal squamous epithelium, whereas acetowhite areas that stain yellow are more likely to be low-grade dysplasia. Areas that remain unstained despite application are more likely to be highly dysplastic tissue if they are within an area that was already abnormal with the acetowhite examination (Figure 29-6).

5. **Endocervical curettage (ECC):** The ECC is performed using an endocervical curette in a mini dilation-and-curettage fashion. Take care to sample only tissue from the cervical canal. Accidental sampling of the ectocervical cells can cause a false positive ECC, which has significant implications for treatment. The specimen is collected with both the curette and a Cytobrush. Swish the curette into a formalin container, and cut the brush tip off into the formalin. Send the specimen for pathologic evaluation.

6. **Cervical biopsy:** Select one to two biopsy sites of the most abnormal appearing areas. Spray on topical anesthetic if available. Position the jaws of the biopsy forceps to optimize the removal of a small piece of ectocervix about 3 mm deep. Hook the spur on the base of the biopsy tip into the cervix at the base of the lesion. Adjust the depth of the biopsy by changing the angle of the forceps relative to the cervical surface and changing the degree of opening of the biopsy tip. The more open the bite when first applied to the cervix, the deeper the bite into the tissue (Figure 29-7). Remove the sample without opening the forceps until it is over the formalin container, and send the biopsy for evaluation. When the biopsy is complete, apply Monsel's solution to obtain hemostasis. Use a dry swab for initial pressure, then quickly apply the Monsel's to the bleeding area before too much blood covers the open vessels. Several rounds of Monsel's application often are required.

7. **Post-procedure:** Remove any blood from the vaginal vault with large swabs, and remove the speculum. Provide the patient with a perineal pad to wear because spotting is likely. Instruct the patient to avoid tampons and intercourse for the next 10 to 14 days. Provide written post-procedure instructions and a clear follow-up plan to review the pathology with the patient.

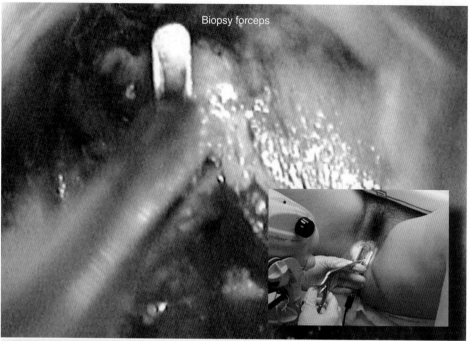

FIGURE 29-7. Cervical biopsy.

ICD-9 CODES

180.9   Cervical neoplasm, malignant (excludes carcinoma in situ)
078.11 Condyloma acuminatum
219.0   Benign neoplasm, cervix
233.1   Ca in situ, cervix
616.0   Cervicitis
622.8   Nabothian cyst
616.10 Vaginitis
622.0   Cervical ectropion
622.0   Cervical erosion/ulcer
622.1   Cervical erosion/ulcer
622.11 CIN I
622.12 CIN II
622.2   Cervical leukoplakia
622.4   Cervical stenosis
622.7   Cervical polyp
622.8   Cervical atrophy
623.0   Dysplasia, vagina
623.1   Vaginal leukoplakia
623.5   Vaginal leukorrhea
623.7   Vaginal polyp
623.8   Vaginal cyst
624.01 Vulvar dystrophy, VIN I
624.0   Vulvar dystrophy, VIN II
624.1   Vulvar atrophy
624.6   Vulvar or labial polyp
795.xx Abnormal Pap (requires five digits for specificity; see Pap smear for details)

Chapter 30

Loop Electrosurgical Excision Procedure (LEEP)

COMMON INDICATIONS

A loop electrosurgical excision procedure (LEEP) is performed to remove high-grade dysplasia (CIN II and CIN III) from the cervix in women older than age 20 and affected by the persistent human papillomavirus disease. The LEEP is also indicated for diagnostic tissue sampling for an unsatisfactory colposcopy or for the removal of visible acetowhite lesions within the endocervical canal. The LEEP is performed to remove these abnormal areas and to provide a pathologic sample in documenting margins from the excision.

EQUIPMENT

The basic equipment for the LEEP includes the base electrosurgery unit, a grounding pad, the LEEP handle, a fine-wire loop tip, and a ball tip for cautery (Figure 30-1). The procedure should be performed with an insulated speculum to reduce the risk of inadvertent electrical arcing from the loop wire tip.

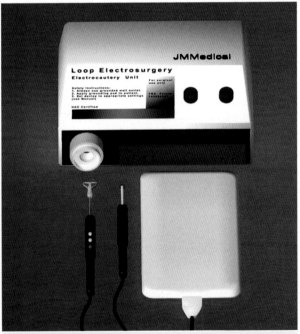

FIGURE 30-1. Equipment.

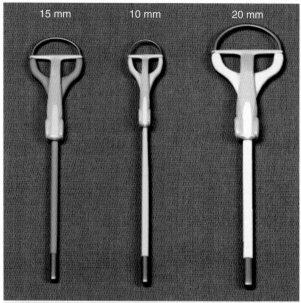

FIGURE 30-2. Common loop-wire sizes.

KEY STEPS

1. **Preparation:** Place the patient in the lithotomy position, place a grounding pad on the patient's thigh, and connect the pad to the LEEP base unit. Connect the LEEP handle to the base unit, and insert the desired loop wire into the end of the LEEP handle (Figure 30-2). Insert an insulated vaginal speculum, and clearly visualize the cervix. Connect the smoke evacuation hose to the speculum to ensure clear visibility during the procedure.

2. **Anesthesia:** Apply 5% acetic acid to the cervix. Identify the margins of the dysplastic tissue to be removed. Lidocaine with epinephrine is injected in 1-cc amounts circumferentially around the planned excision area to provide a complete field block of the area to be excised. These injections should be done at 12 o'clock, 2 o'clock, 4 o'clock, 6 o'clock, 8 o'clock, and 10 o'clock positions. Starting with the lower injections (at 4 o'clock, 6 o'clock, and 8 o'clock positions) and injecting slightly larger volumes will tilt the cervix into a more favorable aspect for the rest of the procedure. Inject 1 cc of anesthetic at 6 o'clock and 12 o'clock positions just at the opening of the os, a full cm deep angled away from the os, if a top-hat excision is planned (Figure 30-3).

3. **Safety considerations:** All transfers of the LEEP instruments in and out of the vaginal canal must be done carefully to avoid accidental contact with the sidewalls with a potentially hot instrument tip. To aid in this safety measure, always rest any of the instruments on the lower blade of the speculum, especially if you are taking your eyes off of the field or the scope during instrument transfers (Figure 30-4).

4. **Selection of loop wire:** Excisions of the transformation zone are performed with the semi-circular loop tip, and top-hat excisions are performed with either a square loop device or a smaller semicircular 10-mm loop tip. The loop wire should be large enough to remove the bulk of the lesion and the outer aspect of the endocervical canal in one pass (Figure 30-5). A 15-mm loop for the initial pass will suffice for most excisions. Reserve the 20-mm loops for larger lesions.

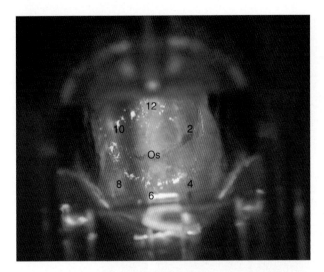

FIGURE 30-3. Injection sites for an intracervical block.

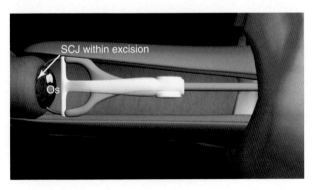

FIGURE 30-4. Resting syringe and needle on lower speculum blade during transfers.

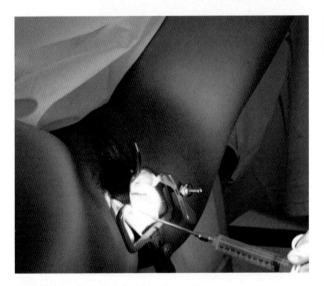

FIGURE 30-5. Excision of squamocolumnar junction in the first pass.

FIGURE 30-6. First LEEP pass with the CUT mode.

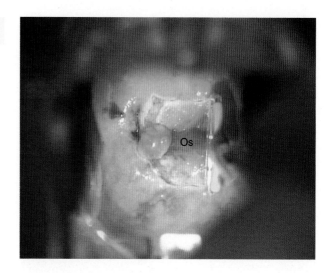

5. **Excision:** The initial pass of the excision should include the entire transformation zone above and below the os. Identify the planned surgical margins. The operator must ensure that the CUT button is selected on the LEEP handle and then stabilize the hand holding the instrument. Make several practice passes before activating the CUT button, and then make the actual excision pass over with the os centered in the pass (Figure 30-6). If there is any remaining high-grade dysplastic tissue, secondary and tertiary passes may be required to remove all visible abnormal areas.

6. **Inspection of endocervix:** After the excision is complete, hold pressure on the wound site with a large swab. Remove the swab, and inspect the endocervical canal for any signs of remaining dysplasia in the endocervical canal. If there is acetowhite epithelium (AWE) further in the canal, perform a LEEP-conization or a top-hat procedure with a second pass just over the endocervical canal at a depth of at least 5 mm.

7. **Hemostasis:** After all of the passes are completed, use the electrocautery (COAG or HEMO) mode of the LEEP device and compress with large swabs to obtain hemostasis. First cauterize the deeper aspects of the excision, and work the cautery outward. If the outer margins are first cauterized, the excision involutes, and it becomes more difficult to cauterize the deeper areas. Cauterize any remaining low-grade areas that may be at the margins of the LEEP excision. Apply Monsel's solution to coat the cauterized area to enhance hemostasis (Figure 30-7). When adequate hemostasis is obtained, carefully remove the speculum.

8. **Follow-up:** The patient should return in 2 weeks for examination to ensure that the excision site is healing well, to review the pathology, and to follow the surveillance plan.

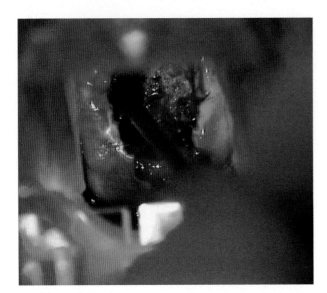

FIGURE 30-7. Cautery of base of excision using the COAG or HEMO mode.

ICD-9 CODES

180.9   Cervical cancer
233.1   CIN 3 (severe dysplasia, ca-in-situ)
622.11   CIN 1
622.12   CIN 2
795.04   High-grade squamous intraepithelial lesion

Chapter 31

Paracervical Block

COMMON INDICATIONS

Paracervical blocks can provide excellent anesthesia for procedures that involve cervical dilation, uterine aspiration, or instrumentation of the uterus. The paracervical block is not recommended for loop electrosurgical excision procedure (LEEP) procedures because it may not be as dense on the surface of the cervix as an intracervical block (Figure 31-1).

EQUIPMENT

The equipment needed for the block includes a local anesthetic such as 2% lidocaine, a 10-cc syringe, a needle extender, an 18-gauge needle, and a 1¼-inch, 27-gauge needle. Draw up 8 cc of lidocaine into the syringe using the 18-gauge needle. Remove the needle, and attach the 27-gauge needle to the needle extender (Figure 31-2).

KEY STEPS

1. **Preparation:** Place the patient in the lithotomy position, insert the speculum, and visualize the entire cervix. Clean off any mucus or discharge from around the apex of the vaginal vault.

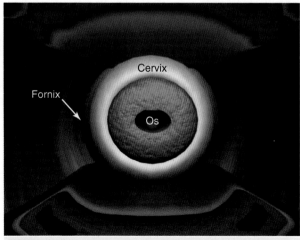

FIGURE 31-1. Anatomy.

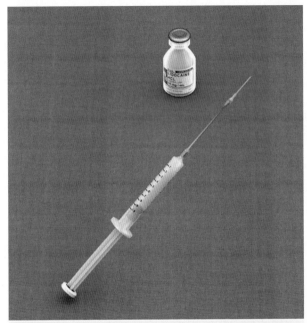

FIGURE 31-2. Equipment.

2. **Anesthesia:**
- *Four-point technique:* Identify the cervical-vaginal junction or the fornix. The injections will be performed at this junction. First, inject at the 10 o'clock position. Use the needle and extender to move the cervix into position to ensure placement of the needle on the lateral margin of the cervix at the fornix. Aspirate before injecting to avoid direct intravascular injection. Inject 2 cc of lidocaine at each site. Then perform injections at 8 o'clock, 2 o'clock, and 4 o'clock positions. Use a large swab to adjust the cervical position, and aid in visualizing each injection site (Figure 31-3A, B).
- *Two-point technique:* Identify the midpoint between the os and the lateral margin of the cervix on each side of the os. Inject at 9 o'clock and 3 o'clock positions deep into the cervix approximately 3 cm. Inject 5 to 10 cc on each side (Figure 31-4).

3. **Testing of block:** Approximately 3 to 5 minutes after the injections are completed, test the cervix to see whether the patient has sharp sensation. The block is complete when sharp sensation is absent.

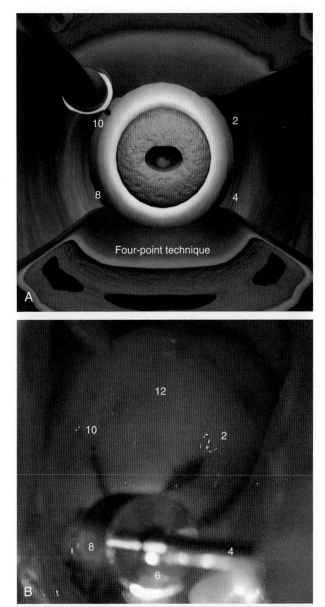

FIGURE 31-3. A-B. Four-point technique: injection sites.

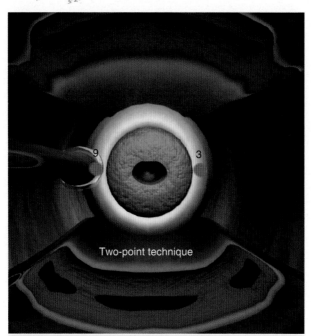

FIGURE 31-4. Two-point technique: injection sites.

ICD-190 CODES

No ICD-9 codes are associated with this procedure

Chapter 32

Uterine Aspiration

COMMON INDICATIONS

Uterine aspiration is performed to manage incomplete or missed abortions during the first trimester of pregnancy. Dilation and curettage (D & C) can be performed as an office procedure or in a same day surgery setting, depending on the gestational age of the pregnancy and patient preference. Mild oral sedation with a paracervical block will provide adequate pain control in the office setting for most patients. Medications to manage hemorrhage such as pitocin, Methergine, or misoprostol should be available in case they are needed.

EQUIPMENT

The instruments needed for the procedure are a tenaculum, a uterine sound, a set of cervical dilators, a flexible plastic suction curette attached to a suction device, and a sharp curette (Figure 32-1). To perform the paracervical block, refer to Chapter 31.

KEY STEPS

1. **Preparation:** Place the patient in the lithotomy position. Cleanse the perineum, vulva, vagina, and cervix with an antiseptic solution. Drape the perineum, leaving access to the vagina and cervix for the procedure. Determine the position of the patient's uterus by performing a bimanual examination. Insert a weighted speculum or a bivalve speculum, depending on the patient's anatomy (Figure 32-2). The cervix must be clearly visible to perform the procedure.

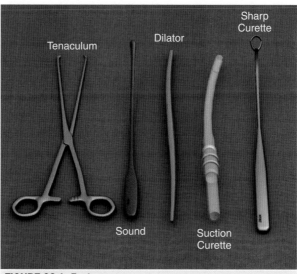

FIGURE 32-1. Equipment.

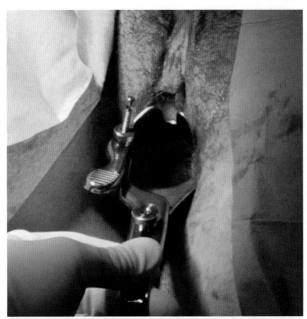

FIGURE 32-2. Visualization of the cervix.

2. **Sounding the uterus:** When adequate anesthesia is obtained, grasp the anterior cervix horizontally with a tenaculum. Insert the uterine sound into the os, and apply gentle pressure until the internal os dilates and the sound enters the uterine cavity. Note the measurement of the internal uterine length by identifying the insertion depth from the external os on the sound. Use this depth as the maximum insertion length of any instrument during the procedure (Figure 32-3).

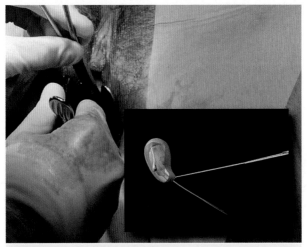

FIGURE 32-3. Sounding of the uterus.

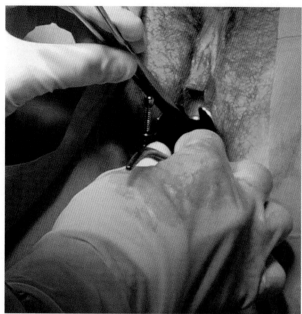

FIGURE 32-4. Dilation of the os with progressive dilator insertion.

3. **Dilation of the os:** If the os is completely closed, start with a 3-mm dilator, and pass the dilator through the internal os, never exceeding the depth of the uterine sound measurement. Gradually increase the dilator diameter, and dilate the os to the same dilation in millimeters as the patient is in gestational weeks (Figure 32-4). This is a general rule, and often the maximum dilation needed is 9 to 10 mm. For most late first-trimester D & C procedures, this will allow a large enough suction curette to be used to evacuate the uterus efficiently.

4. **Suctioning of endometrial cavity:** When fully dilated, leave the last dilator in place while preparing the plastic suction catheter. Use a curved suction catheter for an anteflexed uterus or straight suction catheter for a retroflexed uterus. Remove the dilator, and insert the suction catheter with the suction off. When in the uterine cavity, activate the suction and begin scraping the sidewalls of the uterine cavity to remove the products of conception (POCs). If an ultrasound was done before the procedure, this will allow the operator to focus attention on the known placental implantation site. If the catheter is filled with chorionic or placental tissue, remove the catheter from the uterine cavity, and allow air to be suctioned into the catheter to move the contents to a collection syringe or filter on the suction machine. Repeat aggressive suctioning of the uterine cavity until no bogginess is noted on any aspect of the endometrial lining. This may require three to four sets of suctioning to complete (Figure 32-5).

5. **Confirming an empty uterus:** To check whether there are any residual POCs, a sharp curette can be used to check the uterine cavity for remnants of the POCs. Observe the level of bleeding, which should be very light after all of the POCs are removed.

6. **Aftercare:** Give the patient pitocin for hemostasis, either 10 units IM or 20 units in a liter of normal saline, if needed. When adequate hemostasis is assured, remove the speculum and drapes. Give a single 50 µg of RhoGAM if the patient is Rh negative and the D & C is performed before 13 weeks of gestation. Use the full dose or 300 µg after 13 weeks.

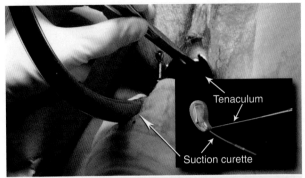

FIGURE 32-5. Aspiration of the uterus.

ICD-9 CODES

622.4   Cervical stenosis
632   Abortion, missed
634.91   Abortion, spontaneous, incomplete
634.92   Abortion, spontaneous, complete
635.90   Abortion, elective
637.90   Abortion, inevitable
637.91   Abortion, incomplete
637.92   Abortion, complete
640.00   Abortion, threatened, unspecified
646.30   Abortion, habitual or recurrent

Ultrasound

Chapter 33

First Trimester Ultrasound

COMMON INDICATIONS

In the first trimester, the transvaginal transducer can be used to diagnose a living embryo, rule in intrauterine pregnancy, rule out multiple gestation, and calculate the gestational age (Figure 33-1).

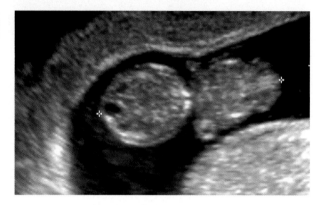

FIGURE 33-1. First trimester intrauterine pregnancy.

KEY STEPS

1. **Position patient and prepare the transducer:** The patient is asked to empty her bladder and place herself in the lithotomy position. Transvaginal ultrasound probes are useful to visualize the pregnancy in the first trimester. (See Chapter 34 on the second and third trimester ultrasound.) Apply a small amount of ultrasound gel to the inside of the probe cover and additional sterile lubricating gel to the tip of the covered transducer (Figure 33-2).

2. **Introduce the transducer:** Gently and slowly insert the transducer 3 to 4 cm in the sagittal plane. Keep the transducer orientation mark on the top (Figure 33-3). Gently move the transducer tip beyond the bladder, and place it near the uterus (Figure 33-4).

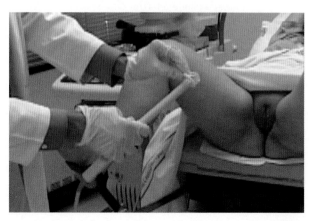

FIGURE 33-2. Place ultrasound gel and cover on transducer.

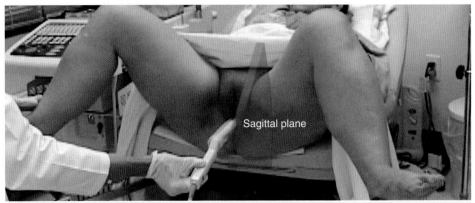

FIGURE 33-3. Insert transducer in the sagittal plane.

3. **Identify the pelvic and fetal anatomy:** Identify the cervix, the endocervical canal, and the decidua if present (Figure 33-5). Keeping the transducer in the sagittal plane, sweep it gently from left to right. Identify the black gestational sac surrounded by white decidua, and locate the fetus (Figure 33-6). Sweep through the entire uterus to rule out multiple gestations.

4. **Fetal cardiac activity:** Use the motion mode to extend a single line of ultrasound signal over time, to document fetal cardiac activity, and to determine the fetal heart rate (Figure 33-7). Failure to identify an intrauterine embryo, gestational sac, or yolk sac can indicate an ectopic gestation. If the quantitative βhCG is appropriately elevated, an empty uterus is an ectopic pregnancy until proven otherwise.

5. **Measuring the crown rump length:** The distance between the top of the fetal head and the end of the sacrum defines the crown rump length. This can accurately determine the fetal age and due date in the first trimester. Slowly rotate the transducer counterclockwise to full transverse plane. Continue rotating the transducer to find the angle that best visualizes the full fetal length. Small adjustments in the pitch of the transducer may be necessary to keep the fetus in view. Unless the fetus is clearly visualized the first time, repeat measurements and determine a mean crown rump length. Report the findings (Figure 33-8).

6. **Ovarian evaluation:** Gently sweep the transducer to the lateral adnexa. First locate one ovary, characterized by the ring of follicles (Figure 33-9). Then sweep to the contralateral side to visualize the other ovary. If an ovarian cyst is noted, appropriate clinical follow-up may be required (Figure 33-10).

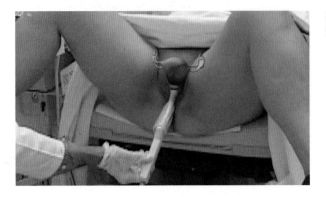

FIGURE 33-4. Place transducer tip near the uterus.

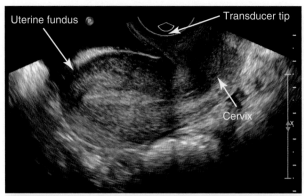

FIGURE 33-5. Identify the uterine fundus and cervix.

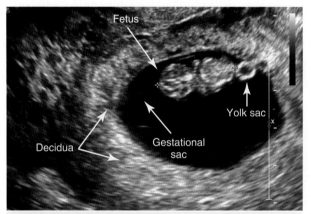

FIGURE 33-6. Fetus, white decidua surrounding black gestational sac, and yolk sac.

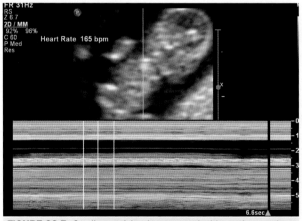

FIGURE 33-7. Cardiac activity documented with motion mode.

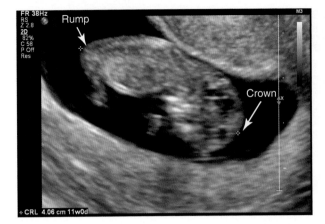

FIGURE 33-8. Measure the crown rump length.

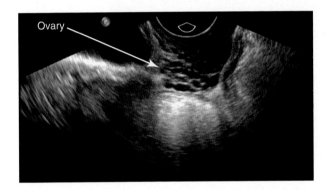

FIGURE 33-9. Visualize both ovaries.

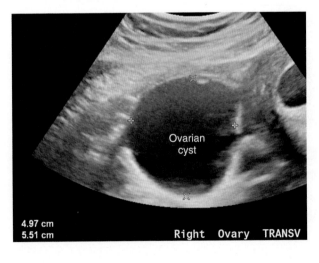

FIGURE 33-10. A simple right ovarian cyst.

ICD-9 CODES

623.8	Vaginal bleeding
630	Hydatidiform mole
632	Missed abortion
633.9	Ectopic pregnancy, unspecified
634.91	Abortion or miscarriage, incomplete, without complications
634.92	Abortion or miscarriage, complete, without complications
640.03	Threatened abortion, antepartum
651.93	Multiple gestation, antepartum

Chapter 34

Basic Second and Third Trimester Obstetric Ultrasound

EQUIPMENT

In the first trimester, the fetus is best visualized with a transvaginal transducer of 5 to 7 MHz. The second and third trimester scans mostly use the 3 to 5 MHz transabdominal transducer (Figure 34-1).

Have the patient lie supine in a comfortable position with a pillow under her head for comfort. Apply transducer gel to her abdomen.

KEY STEPS

1. **Confirm single-living intrauterine pregnancy:** Sweep the entire uterus to check for multiple gestations, and confirm fetal viability by identifying fetal cardiac activity.

2. **Determine presenting part:** To determine the fetal presenting part and orientation, begin the examination in the lower uterine segment with the transducer in the transverse plane (Figure 34-2). Determine the location of the fetal skull. The presence of the fetal skull in the lower uterine segment usually confirms a vertex presentation (Figure 34-3).

3. **Determine orientation:** To determine orientation, visualize the long axis of the fetal spine. After orienting to the fetal spine, you will be three-dimensionally oriented to the fetal position. Visualize fetal extremities or the face to confirm position (Figure 34-4).

4. **Determine placental location:** Scan with the transducer in the sagittal position, slowly scanning from the lower uterine segment to the fundus. The placenta appears as hyperechoic tissue. Calcifications may be observed (Figure 34-5). If the placenta cannot be visualized, it may be located posteriorly, obscured by fetal parts. Note the position of the placenta. If the placenta is near the cervix (placenta previa), it should be noted and followed. Record all findings.

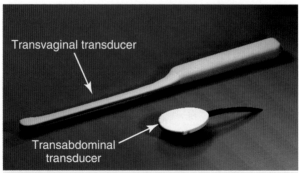

Transvaginal transducer

Transabdominal transducer

FIGURE 34-1. Transvaginal and transabdominal transducers.

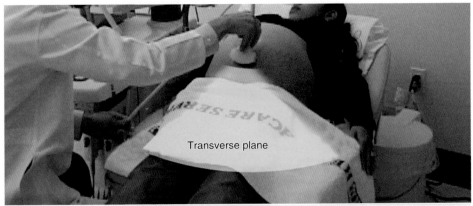

Transverse plane

FIGURE 34-2. Begin scan of the lower uterine segment in the transverse plane.

5. **Measure the amniotic fluid index (AFI):** The AFI is a quantitative evaluation of the amniotic fluid volume. Divide the uterine image into four quadrants centered on the maternal umbilicus (Figure 34-6). Hold the ultrasound transducer in a vertical alignment; keep the transducer perpendicular to the plane of the floor and aligned longitudinally with the mother's spine (Figure 34-7). Starting in one quadrant, identify the pocket of fluid with

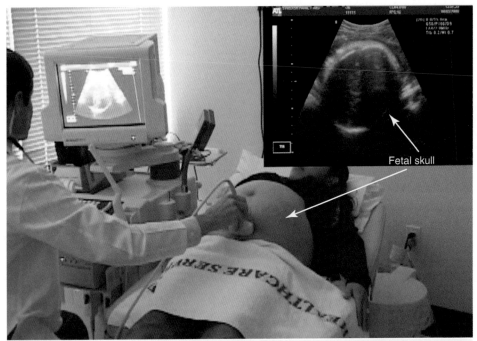

Fetal skull

FIGURE 34-3. Fetal skull in the lower uterus.

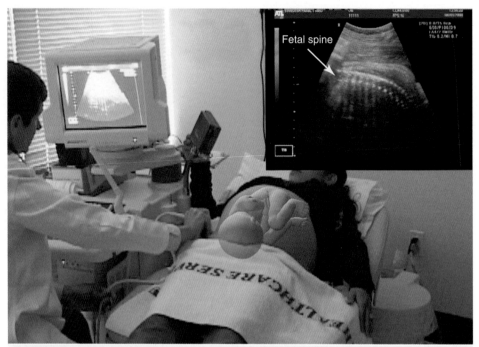

FIGURE 34-4. Orient transducer to the fetal spine.

the largest vertical dimension that is free of fetal parts and cord. Take care to avoid including segments of the umbilical cord in the measurement. Coiled cord can fill the space and sometimes appear to be fluid. Measure the pocket size and record the findings. Repeat this procedure in each quadrant. Sum the measured depth of all four quadrants to determine the AFI. A normal AFI is between 8 and 20 cm (Figure 34-8).

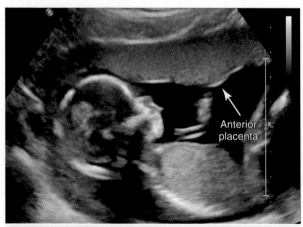

FIGURE 34-5. Anterior placenta.

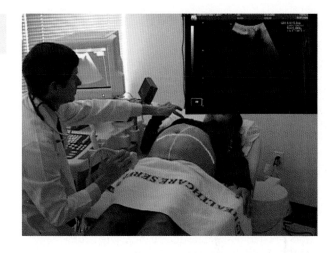

FIGURE 34-6. To measure the AFI, divide the abdomen into four quadrants.

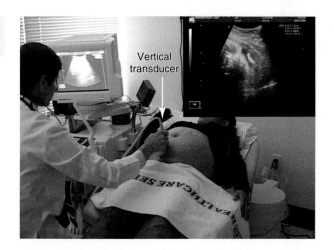

FIGURE 34-7. Keep transducer vertical to measure depth of the fluid pocket.

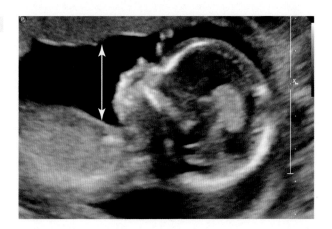

FIGURE 34-8. Measuring the AFI.

ICD-9 CODES

623.8	Vaginal bleeding
630	Hydatidiform mole
634.91	Abortion or miscarriage, incomplete, without complications
634.92	Abortion or miscarriage, complete, without complications
640.03	Threatened abortion, antepartum
641.03	Placenta previa without hemorrhage, antepartum
641.03	Placenta previa with hemorrhage, antepartum
641.21	Placental abruption, delivered
641.23	Placental abruption, antepartum
644.20	Preterm labor
644.21	Preterm labor, delivered
645.13	Postterm pregnancy (40-42 weeks), antepartum
645.23	Prolonged pregnancy (>42 weeks), antepartum
646.83	Uterine size/date discrepancy, antepartum
651.93	Multiple gestation, antepartum
656.53	Intrauterine growth retardation
656.63	Fetal macrosomia, antepartum
657.3	Polyhydramnios, antepartum
658.3	Oligohydramnios, antepartum

Chapter 35

Measurement of Cervical Length

COMMON INDICATIONS

Cervical length can be more reliably and reproducibly determined by a transvaginal ultrasound and can help identify pregnancies at a higher risk of preterm delivery.

KEY STEPS

1. **Prepare the patient and the transducer:** The patient should be asked to empty her bladder immediately preceding the procedure. The transvaginal transducer is topped with ultrasound gel and covered with a sterile sheath, and then topped with sterile lubricant. (See Figure 2 in Chapter 33: First Trimester Ultrasound.) The transducer is gently and slowly introduced through the introitus in the sagittal plane. (See Figure 3 in Chapter 33: First Trimester Ultrasound.) After slightly compressing the anterior cervical lip, withdraw the transducer so that the cervix is not visibly compressed.

2. **Identify the cervical anatomy:** Visualize the cervical canal, the internal and external os, and the fetal presenting part (Figure 35-1).

3. **Measuring the cervical length:** Take three measurements in the long axis of the closed cervical length over the course of 3 minutes, from internal to external os. If the cervix is significantly curved, the length will need to be estimated by making two or three lines from the curve (Figure 35-2).

4. **Document the average finding:** The normal cervical length in the second and third trimesters is 2.5 cm or more. Document funneling (Figures 35-3 and 35-4) or dilation (Figure 35-5) if present.

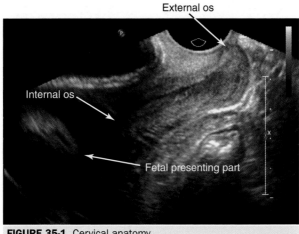

FIGURE 35-1. Cervical anatomy.

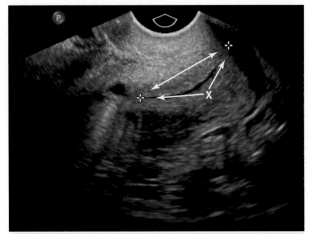

FIGURE 35-2. Measuring cervical length.

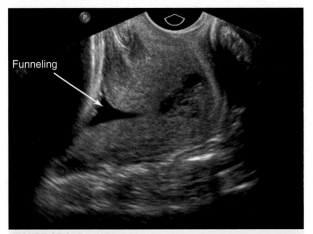

Funneling

FIGURE 35-3. Funneling.

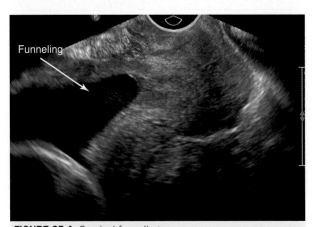

Funneling

FIGURE 35-4. Cervical funneling.

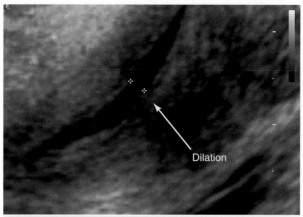

FIGURE 35-5. Dilation of the cervical canal.

ICD-9 CODES

2009 ICD-9-CM Diagnosis Code 649.73
Cervical shortening, antepartum condition or complication
2010 ICD-9-CM Diagnosis Code 644.03
Threatened premature labor antepartum
2010 ICD-9-CM Diagnosis Code 644.13
Other threatened labor antepartum
2010 ICD-9-CM Diagnosis Code V23.41
Supervision of high-risk pregnancy with history of pre-term labor

Urgent/Hospital Care

Chapter 36

Lumbar Puncture

COMMON INDICATIONS

Lumbar puncture is a common procedure used in the evaluation of cerebrospinal fluid (CSF) and central nervous system (CNS) pressure. The most common indication for the procedure is to rule out CNS infections such as meningitis or encephalitis. The procedure is performed in adults and children.

EQUIPMENT

The equipment for performing a lumbar puncture is packaged in a complete instrument tray that includes a preparation kit, an anesthetic, a spinal needle, an optional pressure catheter system, and collection tubes labeled to indicate the order of the fluid withdrawn (Figure 36-1).

KEY STEPS

1. **Anatomic landmarks:** Place the patient in the flexed lateral decubitus position. Palpate the iliac crest and the lumbar spines at the midline. The iliac crest serves as the landmark that marks the interspace between the third and fourth lumbar (L3, L4) vertebrae. Mark this interspace (Figure 36-2).

2. **Skin cleansing and anesthesia:** Cleanse the skin with an antiseptic solution. Drape the skin with the fenestrated drape to maintain a sterile field. Anesthetize the skin and deep connective tissue with 1% lidocaine (Figure 36-3).

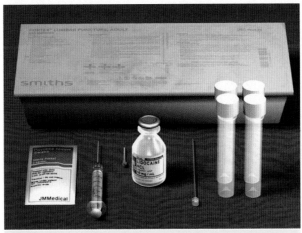

FIGURE 36-1. Lumbar puncture tray with essential contents.

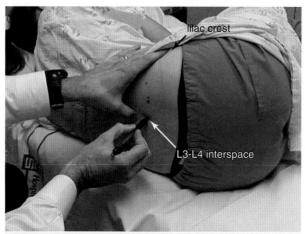

FIGURE 36-2. Anatomic landmarks for lumbar puncture.

3. **Needle insertion:** Insert a 21-gauge spinal needle through the interosseous ligament into the intervertebral space. The needle is advanced toward the umbilicus at a 30° angle in the caudad direction between the L3 and L4 vertebrae (Figure 36-4). Remove the obturator to check for spinal fluid flow if one senses that the needle may have entered the dural space. Usually a slight "pop" is felt when the spinal canal is entered (Figure 36-5). When the canal is entered, the obturator is removed, and the spinal fluid is allowed to flow out into the collection tube. If a CSF pressure measure-ment is desired, attach the Luer-Lock connector and the pressure column. Hold the column vertically, and allow the spinal fluid to rise up the column until the fluid is at a stable level. There may be a slight respiratory variation of this level; use the lowest level as the true CSF pressure.

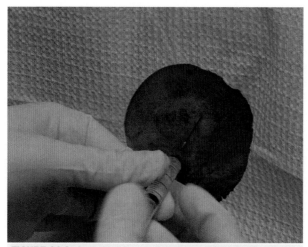

FIGURE 36-3. Anesthetizing track between L3 and L4.

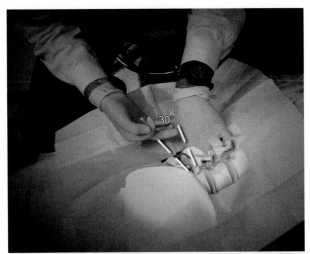

FIGURE 36-4. Needle insertion at appropriate angle to enter between spinous processes.

4. **Fluid collection:** Normally three to four tubes with 1 to 3 cc of fluid are collected and sequentially labeled for CSF studies (Figure 36-6).

5. **Removal of needle:** After the collection of fluid is complete, replace the obturator, and remove the needle from the spinal canal. Cover the site with a simple adhesive dressing.

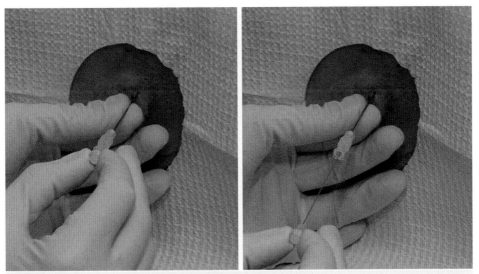

FIGURE 36-5. Entry into spinal canal followed by obturator removal.

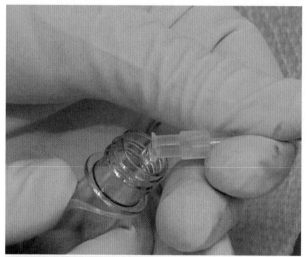

FIGURE 36-6. Collection of CSF.

ICD-9 CODES

322.9   Suspected meningitis
852.00   Subarachnoid hemorrhage
348.2   Pseudotumor cerebri
357.0   Guillain-Barré syndrome
340   Multiple sclerosis
710.0   Systemic lupus erythematosus (SLE)
239.7   Meningeal carcinoma

Chapter 37

Thoracentesis

COMMON INDICATIONS

Thoracentesis is performed to sample or remove fluid that is in the pleural space for both diagnostic and therapeutic purposes. Fluid removed from the chest cavity should be evaluated with red and white cell counts, Gram stains, cultures, chemical markers such as lactate dehydrogenase (also referred to as LDH), protein, and glucose, and cytology studies.

EQUIPMENT

A thoracentesis tray contains Betadine for cleansing the skin, a fenestrated drape, a local anesthetic, a syringe for the local block and a larger syringe for fluid aspiration, a thoracentesis catheter or trocar, and tubing to connect to a drainage system (Figure 37-1A). Have vacuum

FIGURE 37-1. A. Thoracentesis tray. B. Shearing the catheter in a needle-over-catheter system.

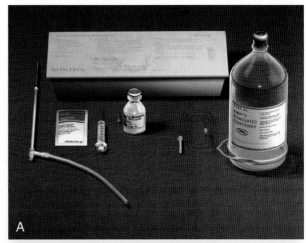

A

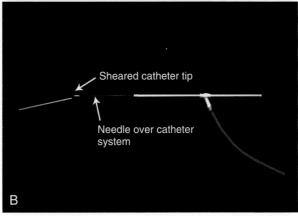

Sheared catheter tip

Needle over catheter system

B

163

bottles or a collection bag available to allow for the drainage of pleural fluid. There are many variations of the kits available, but the two basic catheters are the catheter-over-needle systems and the needle-over-catheter systems. In this case, a needle-over-catheter system is used. In either system, after the needle has been pulled back from the tip of the catheter following insertion into the patient, never re-advance the needle forward or retract the catheter if the needle is still in the patient (Figure 37-1B). This maneuver can shear off the tip of the catheter into the patient's pleural cavity, leaving a foreign body in place that would be difficult to remove.

KEY STEPS

1. **Preparation:** Place the patient in the sitting position with arms resting on a tray table with a pillow for comfort. Determine the level of the pleural effusion by auscultation and percussion. An ultrasound can be used if any question remains about the appropriate level for the thoracentesis. Mark the insertion site well below the top of the effusion but above the twelfth thoracic vertebra (T12), which represents the base of the lung fields. Open the thoracentesis tray, and wear sterile gloves for the procedure. Cleanse the skin area around the insertion site with antiseptic solution, then drape the area with a fenestrated drape (Figure 37-2).

2. **Anesthesia:** The skin should be blocked in a way to allow for the Z technique to be used for the catheter insertion. The marked insertion point should be on a rib, but move the skin upward over the rib during the block so that the insertion point is just above the edge of the rib. Avoid inserting the catheter needle along the lower margin of the rib because

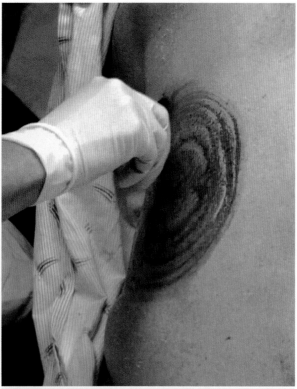

FIGURE 37-2. Preparation.

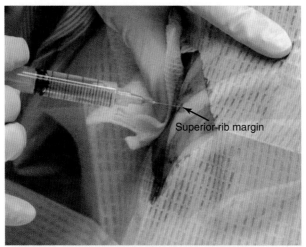

Superior-rib margin

FIGURE 37-3. Local anesthetic along planned catheter trajectory.

it may lacerate an intercostal artery. With lidocaine, create a wheal just below the skin using a 25- to 27-gauge needle for the injection. Advance the syringe in 0.5-cm increments, injecting 0.5 cc of lidocaine every time the needle is advanced (Figure 37-3). After the needle is inserted at least 2 cm, begin to aspirate as the needle is advanced before injecting to see whether the pleural space has been entered. A slight "pop" can be felt when the pleura is entered, and pleural fluid will flow back into the syringe. When in the pleural cavity, slowly inject 1 cc of lidocaine just beyond the entry of the pleural space, then withdraw the needle 3 mm, and again inject 1 cc. This increases the likelihood of adequately blocking the pleura and maximizes patient comfort. Remove the anesthetic syringe and needle, and release the skin tension from the Z maneuver. Drape the area with a fenestrated drape.

3. **Trocar/catheter insertion:** Repeat the Z maneuver to align the skin mark up to the area that was just anesthetized above the rib. Attach the trocar to a closed system using a Luer-Lock valve hub to avoid air intake into the pleural. Insert the trocar through the skin and intercostal muscles. Aspirate using a syringe connected to the closed system as you approach the pleura and when the pleura is penetrated. When in the pleural cavity, advance the catheter forward into the cavity without moving the needle. For trocar-based systems, point the bevel of the trocar downward before advancing the catheter to direct the catheter inferiorly (Figure 37-4).

4. **Removal of pleural fluid:** Connect the tubing to the hub then to the vacuum bottle or collection bag. Open the valve on the hub to allow the flow of pleural fluid to the vacuum bottle. Ideally first draw up some fluid into a 30- or 60-cc syringe through the Luer-Lock Hub for analysis before draining the fluid from the pleural space (Figure 37-5).

5. **Removal of catheter:** When the drainage stops or more than 2 L has been drained, close the hub, and prepare to withdraw the catheter. Do not re-insert the needle; simply pull the catheter out quickly, and release the Z maneuver tension. Apply pressure to the site and a simple adhesive bandage until hemostasis is obtained (Figure 37-6). Send the fluid for analysis, based on the differential for the individual patient.

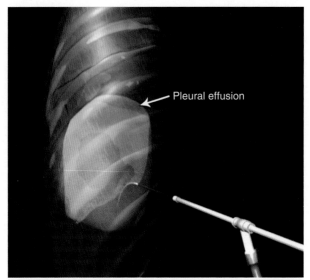

FIGURE 37-4. Ideal position of the catheter downward into the effusion.

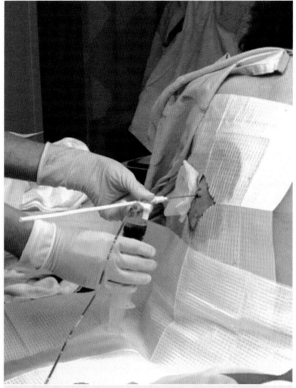

FIGURE 37-5. Obtaining a sample of fluid in the syringe.

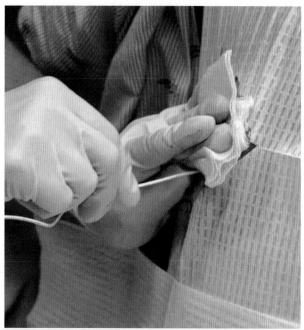

FIGURE 37-6. Removing the thoracentesis catheter.

ICD-9 CODES

511.9	Pleural effusion, unspecified
511.1	Pleural effusion, bacterial
197.2	Pleural effusion, malignant
012.00	Pleural effusion, tuberculous, unspecified
512.8	Pneumothorax, spontaneous, acute or chronic
512.1	Pneumothorax, iatrogenic or postoperative
512.0	Pneumothorax, tension
860.0	Pneumothorax, tension, traumatic

Chapter 38

Paracentesis

COMMON INDICATIONS

Paracentesis is performed for diagnostic or therapeutic reasons in patients with ascites. The volume of fluid removed varies by the patient's pathology and the reason for the procedure. For most paracentesis, remove as much volume as possible, although taking off more than 10 L may cause significant volume shifts and hypotension. Patient comfort is paramount, so placing a good anesthetic block is essential.

EQUIPMENT

Paracentesis kits are available, although for large volume paracentesis, a simple IV catheter with connection tubing and vacuum bottles works well for safe drainage of abdominal fluid. A 3¼-in., 16-gauge IV catheter is ideal for drainage of large volumes (Figure 38-1).

KEY STEPS

1. **Preparation:** The insertion site should be selected on or near the midclavicular line in the lower quadrant at the level of the anterior inferior iliac crest (Figure 38-2). In patients with a large amount of fluid and an empty bladder, a midline entry point approximately 5 to 7 cm below the umbilicus is another approach that is acceptable. Using a portable ultrasound to check the planned entry site is ideal if available, but not required in most cases. In patients with malignant effusions with possible adhesion, ultrasound guidance is preferred. Place the patient in a supine position, and cleanse site with antiseptic solution. The area should be covered with a sterile protective drape.

2. **Anesthesia:** Mark the skin to clearly identify where the anesthetic block will be placed. Inject a wheal in the skin, then insert the needle perpendicularly to the abdominal wall through the center of the wheal into the subcutaneous layer where 0.5 cc of solution is

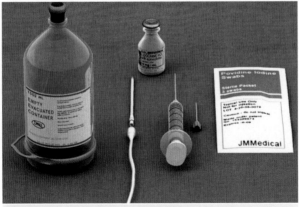

FIGURE 38-1. Equipment for paracentesis.

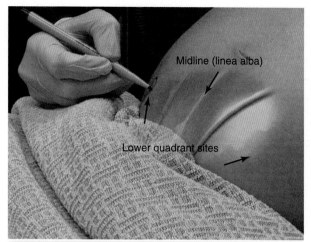

FIGURE 38-2. Selection of site for insertion in lower quadrants or midline sites.

injected. Advance the needle 0.5 cm at a time into the muscle and inject another 0.5 cc. Continue to advance the needle at 0.5-cm increments. Maintain suction on the syringe as the needle is advanced until the abdominal cavity is entered. When ascitic fluid is obtained, the needle is withdrawn several millimeters, and 1 cc of lidocaine is injected at the margin of the peritoneum to numb the peritoneal layer (Figure 38-3).

3. **Catheter insertion:** Insert the drainage catheter down the exact tract of the block, maintaining suction on the syringe attached to the catheter so that it is clear when the peritoneum is penetrated. When the cavity is entered, advance the needle and catheter another 2 mm, then slide the catheter forward off the needle, and remove the needle from the assembly (Figure 38-4). Free flowing fluid should come out of the catheter.

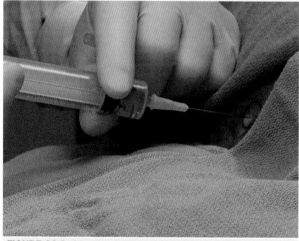

FIGURE 38-3. Anesthesia injected along entry track.

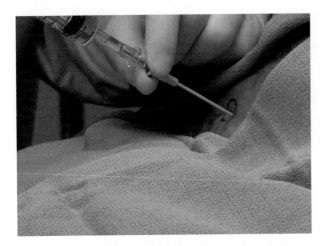

FIGURE 38-4. Advancing catheter over the needle into the peritoneum.

4. **Fluid removal:** Attach the connector tubing to the catheter, then quickly connect it to the collection bottle. A stop cock system or tubing clamp is used to regulate flow when transferring bottles and to avoid spillage (Figure 38-5). If the flow stops before all of the fluid is removed, it is likely that the omentum or bowel wall is occluding the catheter. Close off the suction, and rotate or withdraw the catheter a few millimeters to free the blockage.

5. **Dressing:** At the conclusion of the procedure, remove the catheter. A bulky dressing should be applied over the wound if there is further fluid leak.

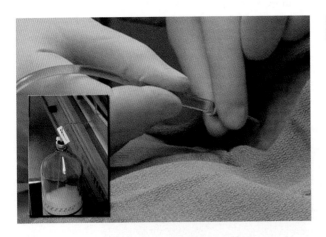

FIGURE 38-5. Connecting tubing to the catheter hub.

ICD-9 CODES

789.5	Ascites
197.6	Ascites, malignant
428.0	Ascites, cardiac
457.8	Ascites, chylous
014.0	Ascites, tuberculous
567.23	Spontaneous bacterial peritonitis

Gastroenterology Procedures

Chapter 39

Anoscopy

COMMON INDICATIONS

Anoscopy can be used to visualize the anal canal and evaluate anorectal symptoms such as pain or bleeding (Figure 39-1).

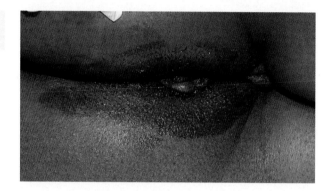

FIGURE 39-1. Anal pathology can be evaluated with an anoscopy.

KEY STEPS

1. **Position patient:** Place the patient in a lateral decubitus position with the knees flexed toward the chest. Hold the buttocks apart and visually inspect the external anatomy.
2. **Digital examination:** After helping the patient relax, lubricate the examining finger and gently perform a digital rectal exam, palpating the anal canal for tone, masses, or tenderness.
3. **Insert anoscope:** Lubricate the anoscope and the central guide plug, and slowly insert the anoscope through the anus (Figure 39-2).

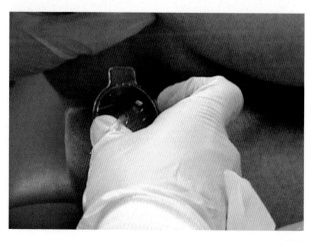

FIGURE 39-2. Gently insert lubricated anoscope.

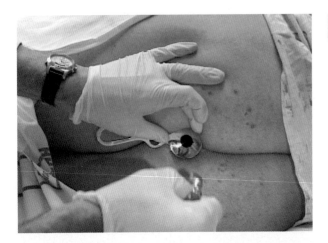

FIGURE 39-3. Remove central guide.

4. **Remove central guide:** After the anoscope is completely inserted, remove the central guide, and place it into a container for soiled instruments (Figure 39-3).

5. **Inspect mucosa:** Slowly rotate the scope as it is withdrawn, and inspect the entire mucosa, looking for mass lesions, hemorrhoids, or fissures (Figure 39-4). Masses or polyps visible through the anoscope may be sampled using a small biopsy forceps.

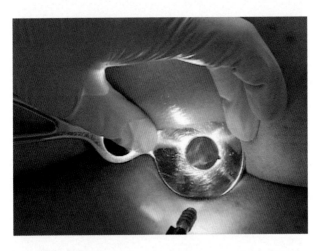

FIGURE 39-4. Rotate the anoscope while withdrawing to visualize entire anus.

ICD-9 CODES

154.1	Cancer, rectum
154.2	Cancer, anus
173.5	Primary malignant lesion, anus, perianal, or gluteal region
198.2	Secondary malignant lesion, anus, perianal, or gluteal region
211.4	Benign neoplasm, colon
455.0	Internal hemorrhoids
216.5	Benign lesion, anus, perianal, or gluteal region
232.5	Carcinoma in situ, anus, perianal, or gluteal region
238.2	Lesion of uncertain behavior, anus, perianal, or gluteal region

239.2   Unspecified lesion, anus, perianal, or gluteal region
455.1   Internal hemorrhoid, thrombosed
455.2   Internal hemorrhoid, bleeding
455.3   External hemorrhoid
455.9   Hemorrhoidal skin tags
555.1   Crohn's disease: colon
556.9   Ulcerative colitis
558.1   Radiation colitis
558.9   Colitis, nonspecific
564.0   Constipation
564.1   Irritable colon
565.0   Anal fissure
565.1   Fistula
566.0   Perirectal abscess
Perianal abscess
Ischiorectal abscess
Intersphincteric abscess
569.0   Anal polyp
569.3   Anal hemorrhage
569.42 Anal pain
698.0   Pruritus ani
787.6   Stool incontinence
787.99 Tenesmus
937.0   Foreign body, anus

Chapter 40

Hemorrhoidectomy

COMMON INDICATIONS

The treatment of thrombosed external hemorrhoids and chronic hemorrhoidal skin tags is best accomplished by local excision (Figure 39-1). A patient can have immediate relief of symptoms and the prompt return to normal activities after these excisions. Conservative management leads to prolonged symptoms, and the hemorrhoids recur often.

EQUIPMENT

A minor surgery tray with lidocaine and bupivacaine, iris scissors, curved hemostats, and gauze are all that is required for treatment (Figure 40-1).

KEY STEPS

1. **Preparation:** The patient is placed in a left lateral Sims' position (Figure 40-2) with knees flexed upward toward the chest. The rectal area is cleaned with Betadine solution. With an acutely thrombosed hemorrhoid, marked tenderness to palpation is common. Recurrent hemorrhoids are often non-tender and leave only a remnant skin tag. The excision technique is the same in both cases, although fresh clots should be removed from acute hemorrhoids.

2. **Anesthesia:** A local anesthetic of a combination of lidocaine and bupivacaine is used to provide a local block. Inject the base of the hemorrhoid around all aspects to ensure complete anesthesia. Injecting the hemorrhoid itself is not necessary if the base is anesthetized. Perform a single deep injection 1 cm deep to the base of an acute hemorrhoid

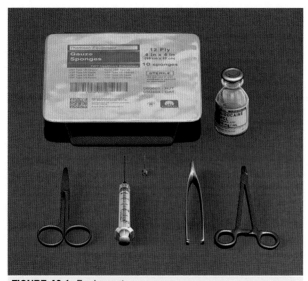

FIGURE 40-1. Equipment.

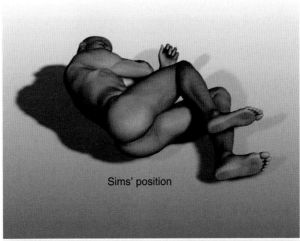

Sims' position

FIGURE 40-2. Positioning the patient for procedure.

to allow for the extraction of any clot within the lesion. Ensure that the central aspect of the hemorrhoid is anesthetized because it is the most common area for failure of the block (Figure 40-3).

3. **Excision of hemorrhoids:** When the anesthesia is complete and allowed to take effect, test the hemorrhoid for sensation. When anesthetized, clamp the hemorrhoid, and excise the hemorrhoid at its base with the iris scissors, cutting an ellipse toward the center of the rectum (Figure 40-4). Spread open the base of the hemorrhoid with hemostats, and express any old clot (Figure 40-5). In acutely thrombosed hemorrhoids, the extraction of clots is critical for relieving symptoms. Usually there is minimal bleeding, and the wound can be left open, allowing for drainage while it is healing.

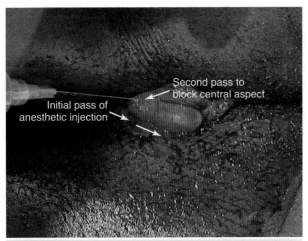

Second pass to block central aspect

Initial pass of anesthetic injection

FIGURE 40-3. Local anesthetic injections to block the base of the hemorrhoid.

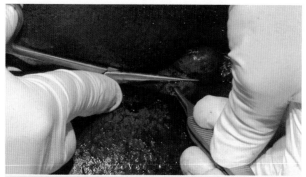

FIGURE 40-4. Excision along the radius of the hemorrhoid toward the anal opening.

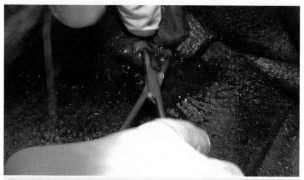

FIGURE 40-5. Exploration to remove clot.

4. **Aftercare:** Place gauze over the anal area, and have the patient dress with snug underwear. Instruct the patient to rinse the area for the next 3 days after any bowel movements. Proper cleansing of the area is important to reduce the risk of postoperative infection.

ICD-9 CODES

4559   Hemorrhoidal tag
455.9   Hemorrhoid tag
455.3   External hemorrhoids
455.4   External hemorrhoids, thrombosed

Chapter 41

Male Bladder Catheterization

COMMON INDICATIONS

Urinary bladder catheterization is an important procedure used to diagnose problems of the urinary tract and to manage fluid balance.

EQUIPMENT

Bladder catheterization equipment can be obtained in sterile kits that contain the sterile catheter, antiseptic solution and cotton balls, lidocaine jelly, and urine collection containers (Figure 41-1).

KEY STEPS

1. **Position and prepare the patient:** Open the kits, put on sterile gloves, and cover the patient with a fenestrated drape (Figure 41-2). Open the antiseptic solution, and pour it onto cotton balls. Thoroughly cleanse the urethral meatus with antiseptic solution (Figure 41-3).

2. **Insert the catheter:** Lubricate the catheter with 2% lidocaine jelly (Figure 41-4). Gently insert the tip of the catheter through the urethra. Pass the entire length of the catheter into

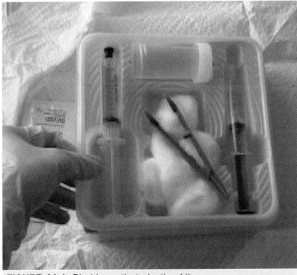

FIGURE 41-1. Bladder catheterization kit.

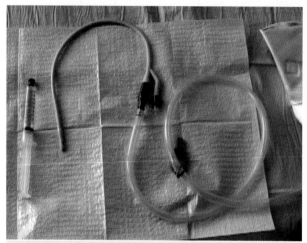

FIGURE 41-2. Open kit and drape patient.

the urethra up to the junction of the inflation port (Figure 41-5). Insert at least 20 cm of the catheter into the urethra to ensure that the tip is fully inside the bladder.

3. **Inflate balloon:** If the catheter is to be left in the bladder, inflate the balloon tip by inject-ing 10 cc of sterile water into the balloon port (Figure 41-6). Gently pull on the catheter to ensure that the balloon is fully inside the bladder and will prevent the catheter from slipping out.

4. **Urine analysis:** Obtain urine in sample containers labeled with the patient's identifying information, and send it to the laboratory for analysis (Figure 41-7).

5. **Catheter removal:** When removing the catheter, first deflate the balloon by withdrawing the 10 cc of water from the balloon port, then slowly slide the catheter out of the bladder.

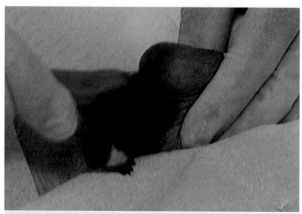

FIGURE 41-3. Cleanse urethral meatus.

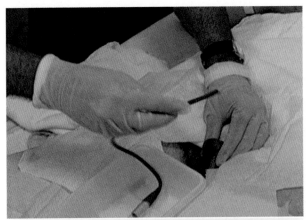

FIGURE 41-4. Lubricate the catheter with 2% lidocaine jelly.

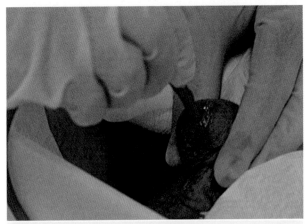

FIGURE 41-5. Gently insert the catheter.

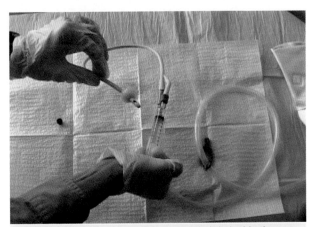

FIGURE 41-6. Inflate the balloon tip (while it is inside the patient's bladder).

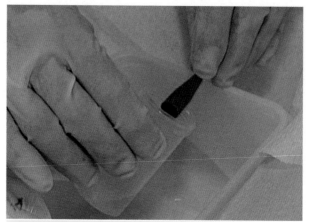

FIGURE 41-7. Collect urine in a specimen cup.

ICD-9 CODES

57.94	Insertion of indwelling urinary catheter
57.95	Replacement of indwelling urinary catheter
96.48	Irrigation of indwelling urinary catheter
97.64	Removal of indwelling urinary catheter

Chapter 42

Female Bladder Catheterization

COMMON INDICATIONS

Urinary bladder catheterization is an important procedure used to diagnose problems of the urinary tract and to manage fluid balance.

EQUIPMENT

Bladder catheterization equipment can be obtained in sterile kits that contain the sterile catheter, antiseptic solution and cotton balls, lidocaine jelly, and urine collection containers (Figure 42-1).

KEY STEPS

1. **Prepare patient and kit:** Place the patient comfortably in the lithotomy position. Open the kit, put on sterile gloves, and cover the patient with a fenestrated drape. The kit can be set up between the patient's legs or on a side table.

2. **Cleanse the urethra:** Open the antiseptic solution, and pour it onto cotton balls. Gently separate the labia with your nondominant hand, and thoroughly cleanse the labia and urethral meatus. Usually three or four antiseptic-soaked cotton balls will be necessary.

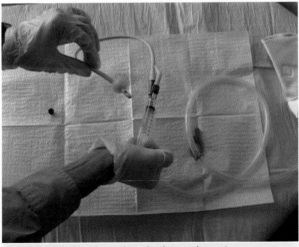

FIGURE 42-1. Bladder catheterization equipment.

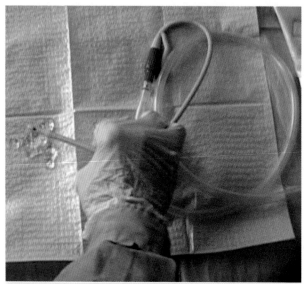

FIGURE 42-2. Lubricate the catheter.

3. **Insert the catheter:** Lubricate the catheter with 2% lidocaine jelly (Figure 42-2). Gently insert the tip of the catheter through the urethra (Figure 42-3). Insert at least 20 cm of the catheter into the urethra to ensure that the tip is fully inside the bladder.

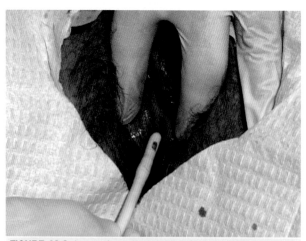

FIGURE 42-3. Insert the catheter through the urethra.

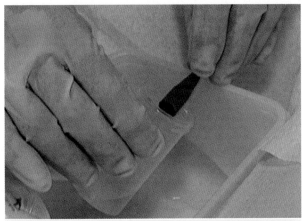

FIGURE 42-4. Collect a urine sample.

4. **Urine sample:** Obtain urine in sample containers labeled with the patient's identifying information, and send it to the lab for an analysis (Figure 42-4).

5. **Inflate the balloon tip:** If the catheter is to be left in the bladder, inflate the balloon tip by injecting 10 cc of sterile water into the balloon port (Figure 42-5). Gently pull on the catheter to ensure that the balloon is fully inside the bladder and will prevent the catheter from slipping out.

6. **Removing the catheter:** When removing the catheter, first deflate the balloon by withdrawing the 10 cc of water from the balloon port, and then slowly slide the catheter out of the bladder.

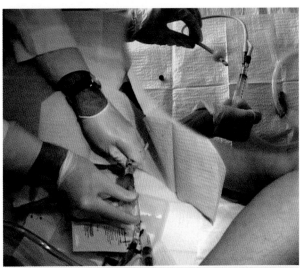

FIGURE 42-5. Inflate the balloon.

ICD-9 CODES

57.94 Insertion of indwelling urinary catheter
57.95 Replacement of indwelling urinary catheter
96.48 Irrigation of indwelling urinary catheter
97.64 Removal of indwelling urinary catheter

Chapter 43

No-Scalpel Vasectomy

COMMON INDICATIONS

The no-scalpel vasectomy is an efficient, nearly bloodless procedure to provide elective sterilization that is safe and effective. The patient should be counseled about the risks of bleeding in the form of scrotal hematomas, infection, and the rare recanalization event.

EQUIPMENT

Use a minor surgical tray with two vasectomy clamps and a dissecting forceps for entering the skin. This sharply pointed forceps is honed to a fine point to puncture and separate the skin for the incisions. Use lidocaine and bupivacaine together to provide a longer block after the procedure (Figure 43-1).

KEY STEPS

1. **Preparation:** Before the procedure, the patient should completely shave the scrotum on the anterior and lateral sides. There is no need to shave the pubic area. Cleanse the skin with an antiseptic solution before draping the patient's genitals so that only the scrotum is exposed (Figure 43-2).

2. **Isolation of the vas:** The most technically challenging portion of a vasectomy is the isolation of the vas. When performing the lateral approach, grasp the vas by pushing the thumb posteriorly at the midline of the scrotum, then isolate the vas laterally with the finger. Push the vas tubule between the index and third fingers with the thumb, and bring the vas to the surface with a lateral rotation movement. When repositioning the vas more laterally and anteriorly, always keep the thumb and middle finger compressed behind the vas to prevent it from slipping back and out of your grasp (Figure 43-3A). If performing a single midline

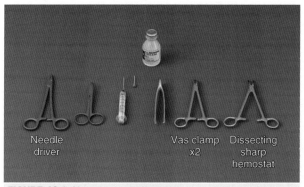

FIGURE 43-1. Vasectomy equipment.

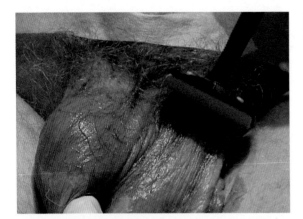

FIGURE 43-2. Shaving of the incision sites (bilateral approach).

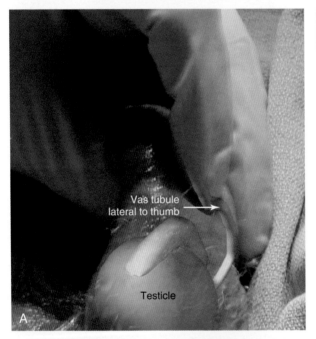

FIGURE 43-3. A-B. Isolation of the vas with thumb, index, and middle fingers.

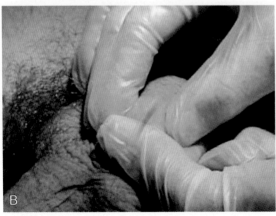

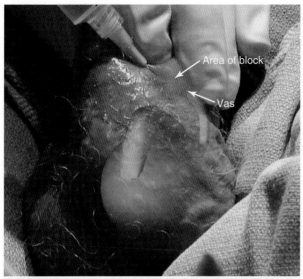

FIGURE 43-4. Block of the vas tubule proximally and distally.

incision, the hand position is different. The index and third fingers lift the vas to the midline moving lateral to medial, while the thumb holds the vas in position during the clamping process after anesthesia is given (Figure 43-3B). When secured, do not relax your grip until the anesthesia and the vas clamp are applied.

3. **Anesthetizing the vas:** Inject a wheal in the scrotal skin over the isolated vas tubule that is held in position by the operator's hand. Anesthetize above and below the area where the tubule will be separated (Figure 43-4). Auto injectors are available to deliver a discrete amount and area of anesthesia to the vas and scrotal skin. After the block is placed, clamp the vas by pushing it into the vas clamp opening using the thumb (Figure 43-5). Ideally do not clamp the vas itself; just grasp the tissue surrounding the vas. This will allow for easier mobilization of the vas tubule from the surrounding fascia.

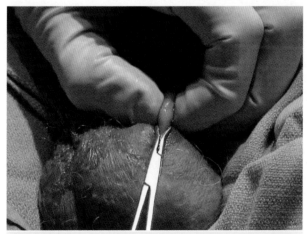

FIGURE 43-5. The vas captured through skin by the vas clamp.

4. **Dissection of the vas:** Use the dissecting forceps to pierce the skin and dissect down to the vas sheath. The vas sheath is then further dissected through the layers of supporting fascia to expose the tubule itself. To release the vas from the scrotum, the fascia layers of the vas can be speared with the sharp dissecting hemostat. The two vasectomy clamps are released and reapplied to the tubule, taking care to grasp only the dissected tubule without any overlying fascia. Release the first clamp only when the second clamp securely holds the vas tubule. This may need to be repeated several times to fully remove the fascia from the tubule. The operator must be very careful not to lose control of the tubule because it may drop into the scrotum and can be more difficult to isolate where the tubule and the skin are actually anesthetized.

5. **Separation of the vas tubule:** When the tubule is freed from the underlying fascia (Figure 43-6), there are several steps for severing the vas and promoting successful scarring of the tubule ends. Remove a segment of the tubule. Cauterize down both sides of the tubule to scar the inner lining of the tubule itself (Figure 43-7). Suture the open ends of each tubule using chromic suture to encourage scarring. The proximal end of the tubule can be allowed to retract down the sheet, and the fascia can be sewn over to further prevent reanastomosis of the tubule. Before the vas is reinserted into the scrotum, hemostasis must be ensured. The most common areas of bleeding are from the vascular structures within the fascia surrounding the vas. These can be cauterized or sutured as needed. When hemostasis is complete, the vas is allowed to fall back into the scrotum. The incision is small enough that sutures are not required.

6. **Completion of procedure:** The procedure is repeated on the opposite side in the same manner. After completion, cover the small incisions with gauze, and have the patient wear an athletic supporter for the next week. Minimal activity is advised for the first 3 days after the procedure.

Dissected tubule

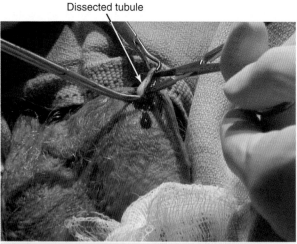

FIGURE 43-6. Dissected vas tubule.

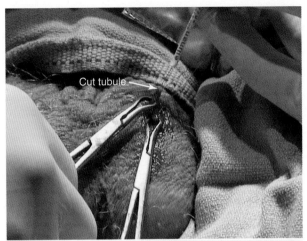

Cut tubule →

FIGURE 43-7. Cautery of the tubule after excision of the segment.

ICD-9 CODES

63.73   Vasectomy
63.7   Vasectomy and ligation of vas deferens

Chapter 44

Bladder Aspiration— Suprapubic Tap

COMMON INDICATIONS

The suprapubic tap provides an excellent option for obtaining a sterile urine sample when a catheterization is not successful. It is most commonly performed in infants but could be done on any patient with a full bladder, requiring a sampling of urine (Figure 44-1).

EQUIPMENT

The equipment needed for a bladder aspiration includes a cleansing solution, a 10-cc syringe, and a 1 in. or greater, 23- to 25-gauge needle.

KEY STEPS

1. **Preparation:** Secure the infant in a frog-leg position to allow for easy access to the suprapubic area. Palpate the bladder, although it may not be palpable in a distressed infant. Cleanse the skin with Betadine, and drape the area around the pubis. Placing a urine bag on the infant is advisable, in case the child urinates during the procedure (Figure 44-2).

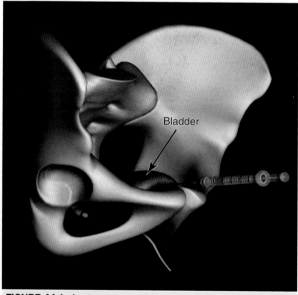

FIGURE 44-1. Anatomy.

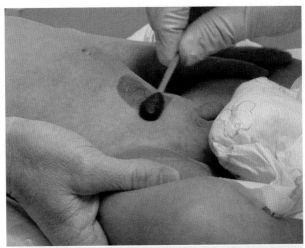

FIGURE 44-2. Positioning of the infant.

2. **Insertion:** Carefully advance a 10-cc syringe with a 23- to 25-gauge needle through the skin just superior to the pubic symphysis. Be sure that the angle of the needle is at 90° with respect to the abdominal wall or slightly caudad to direct it toward the bladder. The syringe plunger is retracted on entry into the subcutaneous layer to create negative pressure. Typically the needle must be inserted 1 to 2 cm to reach the bladder (Figure 44-3).

3. **Aspiration of urine:** When the bladder is entered, urine will be drawn into the syringe (Figure 44-4). When an adequate sample is obtained, the needle is withdrawn and pressure is applied to the site. The specimen is then sent to the laboratory for an analysis.

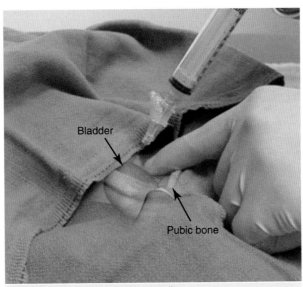

FIGURE 44-3. Insertion of the needle.

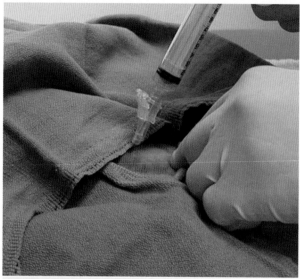

FIGURE 44-4. Aspiration of the bladder.

ICD-9 CODES

599.0 Urinary tract infection, site not specified
780.6 Fever
788.20 Urinary retention or stasis, unspecified
995.91 Sepsis
995.92 Severe sepsis (acute organ dysfunction)

Chapter 45

Circumcision

COMMON INDICATIONS

The three most common elective neonatal circumcision techniques are the Gomco, the Mogen, and the Plastibell techniques. It is important to learn one technique well before attempting to master the other methods. The advantages of each technique are generally equalized by the risks associated with each method. The key anatomic landmarks of the penis are the glans penis, the corona, and the coronal sulcus. During all procedures, care must be taken to avoid dissecting the foreskin beyond the coronal sulcus (Figure 45-1).

EQUIPMENT

For all three procedures, a penile block is performed with a 3-cc syringe, a 27- or 30-gauge needle for injection, and plain lidocaine without epinephrine. Three hemostats, with one being a straight hemostat, suture scissors, a needle driver, and a No. 15 scalpel are essential for performing this procedure (Figure 45-2). Prepare the Gomco clamp by separating its parts and ensuring that they fit properly together and that the bell is large enough to seal against the baseplate. The Mogen should be checked to make sure that the clamp shuts and locks completely and it is not loose. For the third technique, select a Plastibell that will easily fit over the glans; usually a 1.3-cm bell will fit a normal-sized glans. The Plastibell string is extended, and a half surgeon's knot is tied loosely for the first step of the technique.

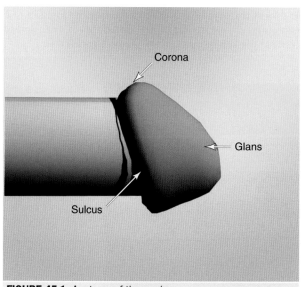

FIGURE 45-1. Anatomy of the penis.

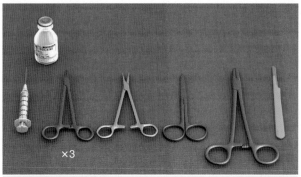

FIGURE 45-2. Equipment.

KEY STEPS

1. **Preparation:** Parents should be instructed not to feed the infant for 2 hours before the procedure. Secure the infant to a padded circumcision board. Cleanse the penis with Betadine solution.

2. **Anesthesia:** Inject 0.3 cc of a local anesthetic at 2 o'clock and 10 o'clock positions and for improved rates of successful blocks, and inject 0.1 cc of a local anesthetic at the base of the frenulum. Always perform the frenulum block in the perpendicular plane to the shaft to avoid injecting into the urethra (Figure 45-3).

3. **Dissection of the foreskin:** When the anesthetic has been in place for 1 to 2 minutes, clamp the tip of the foreskin at 2 o'clock and 10 o'clock positions with hemostats. A third closed straight hemostat is carefully advanced into the opening of the foreskin to coronal sulcus to dissect the adhesions between the glans and the foreskin. Care must be taken not to enter the urethra at any time or pass the tip of the hemostat beyond the proximal end of the glans. Tent the skin as the hemostat is advanced under the foreskin to ensure that the meatus has not been entered. First dissect off the dorsal aspect, then spread the hemostat open, as shown, to sweep the adhesions from the glans (Figure 45-4).

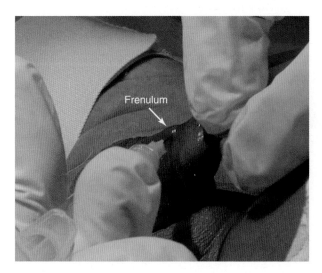

FIGURE 45-3. Anesthesia—frenulum block on the underside of the penis.

Frenulum

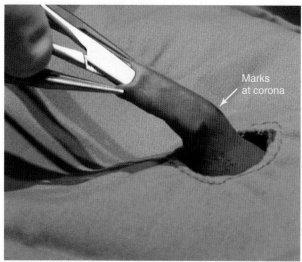

Marks at corona

FIGURE 45-4. Dissection of the foreskin.

4. **Mogen procedure:** After releasing the adhesions, mark the foreskin without tension applied along the arc of the glans about 5 mm distal to the coronal sulcus. Slide the foreskin distally past the tip of the penis, and slide it up to the marked foreskin into the minimally opened Mogen clamp, with the sulcus of the clamp facing the penis (Figure 45-5A). Check that the angle of the clamp matches the angle of the glans. Check to make sure that the glans is not trapped within the foreskin to be excised. Clamp and lock the Mogen clamp. Use a No. 11 or No. 15 blade scalpel to cut away the foreskin from the clamp's outer surface (Figure 45-5B). Remove the clamp after 3 minutes, and carefully open the severed tip of the remnant foreskin. Retract the foreskin behind the glans, and remove any adhesions that may be at the corona of the glans (Figure 45-5C). Check for dehiscence or bleeding.

5. **Gomco technique:** When the entire circumference of the foreskin has been freed, the hemostat is inserted with one tip inside the foreskin along the dorsal surface and clamped for 10 seconds to mark the future midline incision. The clamp should be advanced to only about 5 mm distal to the coronal sulcus (Figure 45-6A). Incise the foreskin to about 5 mm distal to the junction of the coronal sulcus. Carefully dissect the remaining adhesions to allow for a complete retraction of the foreskin back beyond the glans. Place the Gomco bell over the glans under the foreskin layer, and clamp the foreskin over the bell to hold it in place (Figure 45-6B). Pass the baseplate over the bell post, then pull the foreskin up through the baseplate opening, and remove the original hemostat. Using a hemostat or forceps, pull on the mucosal edge of the dorsal slit to make sure that the mucosal apex of the dorsal slit is also above the baseplate. Slide the baseplate forward completely onto the bell. Check the angles of the plate and the bell, and make sure that they align with the angle of the corona (approximately 40°). Slide the rocker arm of the Gomco under the arms of the bell post. Recheck the alignment of the bell and the baseplate. If satisfied with the alignment, secure the rocker to the baseplate with the tightening screw. The groove of the baseplate must align with the pivot under the rocker arm. Leave the clamp in place for 3 to 5 minutes. During that time, the foreskin can be excised from the upper aspect of the bell. Use the very tip of the scalpel to cut and scrape away any remnants of foreskin (Figure 45-6C). Remove the clamp, and carefully peel the foreskin off the bell edge. Check for dehiscence or bleeding.

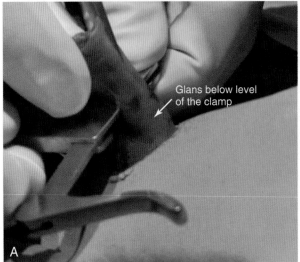

Glans below level
of the clamp

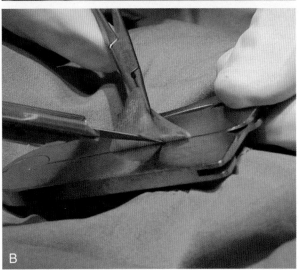

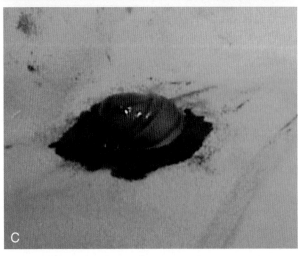

FIGURE 45-5. A. Mogen procedure—clamp application. B. Mogen procedure—cutting distal to the clamp. C. Mogen procedure—removal of adhesions and final appearance.

FIGURE 45-6. A. Gomco technique—midline clamp and incision site. B. Gomco technique—bell clamped within the foreskin before the baseplate application.

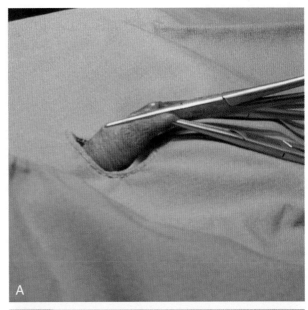

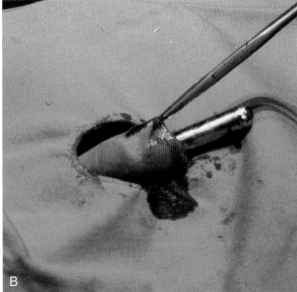

6. **Plastibell technique:** Place the string at the base of the shaft with a relaxed half surgeon's knot in place. Select an appropriate-sized Plastibell. Most infants will accommodate a 1.3-cm bell. Infants with a larger penis should have a 1.4- or 1.5-cm bell. When selecting sizes of bells, err on choosing a larger one. If the bell is too small, it will lead to injury to the glans in the form of pressure ulceration during the healing process after the procedure. When the entire circumference of the foreskin has been

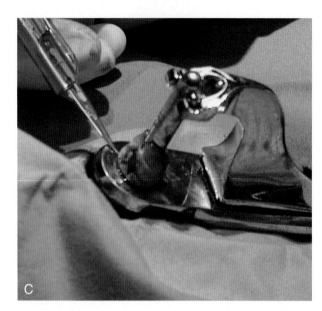

FIGURE 45-6—Cont'd. C. Gomco technique—cutting of foreskin around the bell.

freed, the hemostat is inserted with one tip inside the foreskin along the dorsal surface and clamped for 10 seconds to mark the future midline incision. The clamp should be advanced to only about 5 mm distal to the coronal sulcus. Incise the foreskin to about 5 mm distal to the junction of the coronal sulcus (Figure 45-7A). Carefully dissect the remaining adhesions to allow for a complete retraction of the foreskin back beyond the glans. Pull the foreskin forward to its neutral position with two hemostats, and insert the Plastibell over the glans, as shown. Using the attached hemostats as counterweight on the foreskin and applying forward pressure on the thumb allow the operator to have precise control of the application of the bell while tying the ligature. With the left hand controlling the alignment of the bell and applying traction on the foreskin with the weight of the hemostats, use the right hand to tighten the ligature. Pull the mucosal edge of the dorsal slit to make sure that the mucosal apex of the dorsal slit is distal to the ligature. When the ligature is moderately tight over the bell, release the left hand from the hemostats. Check to make certain that the ligature is in the ligature groove of the bell before proceeding. Tighten the ligature very firmly; the string will not break. Three to four knots are sufficient to secure the knot. Trim the distal portion of the fore-skin at the outer rim of the bell using scissors (Figure 45-7B). Rock the handle of the Plastibell at its base until it breaks free of the ring. Check for hemostasis. Verify that the Plastibell can move up and down about 1 to 2 mm on the glans and that the meatus is not occluded (Figure 45-7A, C).

FIGURE 45-7. A. Plastibell—midline clamp and incision site. B. Plastibell—cutting of foreskin from above ligature. C. Plastibell—one-handed tie of ligature around the bell.

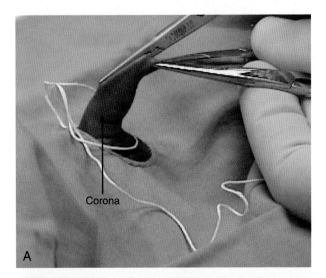

Corona

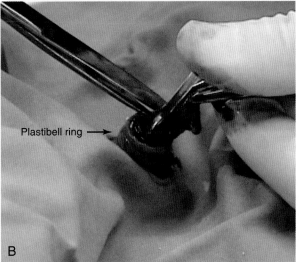

Plastibell ring →

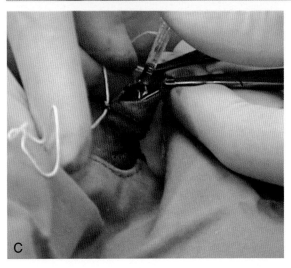

7. **Dressing:** Wrap the tip of the penis with petrolatum gauze. The parents should be given adequate postoperative instructions and a planned follow-up in 1 week to ensure that the appropriate post-circumcision care is being performed.

ICD-9 CODES

V50.2   Circumcision, routine or ritual (in the absence of significant medical indication)
599.6   Urethral obstruction, unspecified

Chapter 46

Penile Biopsy

COMMON INDICATIONS

Penile lesions that are not identifiable as benign or that fail to respond to therapy should be biopsied for a definitive diagnosis and treatment.

EQUIPMENT

A punch biopsy instrument, pick-ups, small iris scissors, and a specimen jar can be used to sample these lesions (Figure 46-1). Lidocaine of 1% without epinephrine, a syringe, and a 27-gauge needle will be necessary for anesthesia. The 5-O absorbable sutures, a needle driver, and suture scissors will be used to close the lesion.

FIGURE 46-1. Equipment.

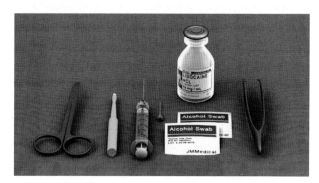

KEY STEPS

1. **Prepare the lesion:** If the patient is not allergic to iodine, clean the lesion with Betadine (Figure 46-2).

FIGURE 46-2. Cleanse the lesion.

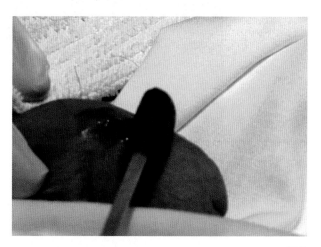

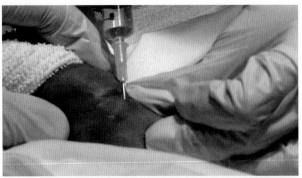

FIGURE 46-3. Inject the local anesthetic.

2. **Topical anesthetic:** Slowly inject 1 to 2 cc of lidocaine under the lesion, elevating it slightly (Figure 46-3). Test the skin to assess adequate anesthesia (Figure 46-4).

3. **Punch biopsy:** Select a suitable-sized punch biopsy instrument to obtain a sufficient sample for diagnosis; 3 mm is usually appropriate. Gently rotate the punch through the dermal layer to a depth of 2 to 3 mm (Figure 46-5). Use a small pick-up to gently lift the sample core, excise it with the tip of a small iris scissors, and place the sample in a labeled specimen jar (Figure 46-6). Hemostasis can usually be achieved with simple pressure.

4. **Suture lesion:** Close the lesion with a single 5-O absorbable suture (Figure 46-7). Provide the patient with warning signs of bleeding or infection, and submit the sample for a pathologic evaluation.

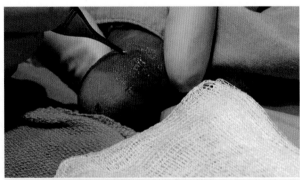

FIGURE 46-4. Test anesthesia.

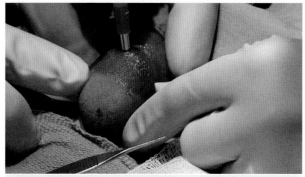

FIGURE 46-5. Obtain the punch biopsy.

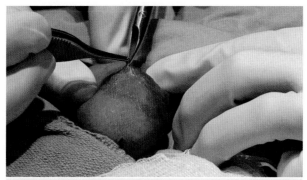

FIGURE 46-6. Free sample with iris scissors.

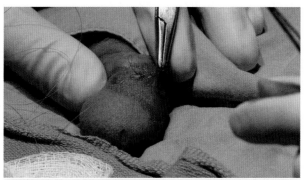

FIGURE 46-7. Suture biopsy site.

ICD-9 CODES

	Neoplasm, skin, penis
187.4	Malignant
198.82	Secondary
232.5	Carcinoma in situ
222.1	Benign
236.6	Benign
239.2	Unspecified

Musculoskeletal Procedures

Chapter 47

Shoulder Injection—
Subacromial Approach

COMMON INDICATIONS

Corticosteroid injections can improve symptoms of osteoarthritis or inflammatory arthritis of the shoulder joint (Figure 47-1).

EQUIPMENT

The equipment includes gloves, povidone-iodine wipes or alcohol wipes, a 1½-in. 25- or 27-gauge needle, an 18-gauge needle and a 10-cc syringe, 1% lidocaine without epinephrine or 0.5% bupivacaine, 20 to 40 mg of methylprednisolone acetate or the equivalent, and an adhesive bandage dressing (Figure 47-2).

KEY STEPS

1. As with all joint injections, sterility must be maintained for any components used in the injection that enters the joint space.
2. Ask the patient to sit comfortably with the arm at rest.

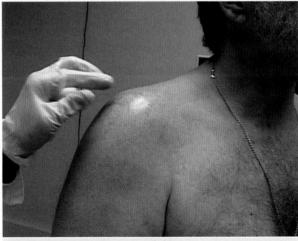

FIGURE 47-1. Shoulder osteoarthritis.

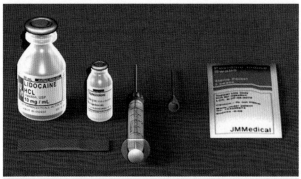

FIGURE 47-2. Equipment.

3. Thoroughly cleanse the shoulder with an antiseptic solution (Figure 47-3). Consider all of the possible diagnoses before proceeding with treatment. Do not inject steroids into a potentially infected shoulder joint.

4. Palpate the bony landmarks, including the head of the humerus, the acromion, and the coracoid process (Figure 47-4).

5. Draw up 3 to 5 cc of 1% lidocaine without epinephrine, or 0.5 % bupivacaine, and 20 to 40 mg of methylprednisolone acetate or the equivalent into a single syringe and mix well by tipping the syringe backward and forward (Figure 47-5).

6. Identify the posterolateral corner of the acromion. Gently insert the needle 1 cm below this point, directed toward the opposite nipple. The needle should encounter little resistance. Do not inject the solution against resistance. Injecting directly into the rotator

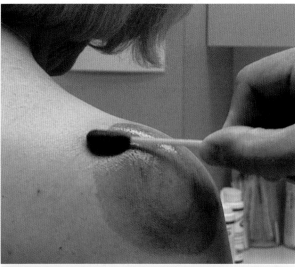

FIGURE 47-3. Thoroughly cleanse the shoulder.

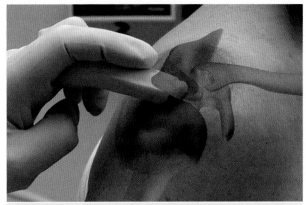

FIGURE 47-4. Palpate the bony landmarks.

cuff can promote a tendon rupture. Aspirate fluid for diagnosis, if necessary, and to ensure proper placement. Slowly inject the corticosteroid solution into the subacromial space (Figure 47-6).

7. Withdraw the needle, and apply gentle pressure to the entry site.
8. Cover the injection site with an adhesive bandage.

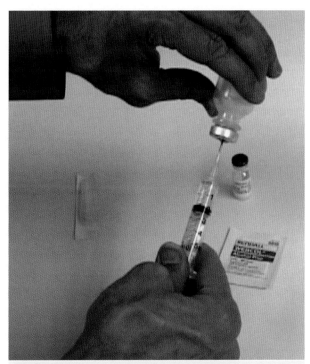

FIGURE 47-5. Draw up the mixture of lidocaine and corticosteroid.

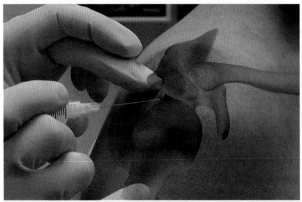

FIGURE 47-6. Inject into the subacromial space.

ICD-9 CODES

274.0 Gouty arthropathy
696.0 Psoriatic arthritis
714.0 Rheumatoid arthritis
715.11 Degenerative joint disease (DJD) shoulder
719.41 Shoulder pain
719.51 Shoulder stiffness
726.10 Bursitis, shoulder
726.10 Rotator cuff syndrome
726.11 Tendinitis shoulder
726.12 Bicipital tendinitis
726.2 Impingement syndrome
727.3 Bursitis
727.82 Calcific tendinitis

Chapter 48

Trochanteric Bursa Injection

COMMON INDICATIONS

Inflammation of the trochanteric bursa leads to chronic, intermittent pain along the lateral hip and tenderness directly over the trochanteric bursa. Corticosteroid injection into the inflamed bursa can effectively improve pain without the systemic side effects of oral antiinflammatory medications. Trochanteric bursitis can mimic other conditions, including disk disease and hip-joint disease, so it is important to consider other diagnoses before proceeding to treatment (Figure 48-1).

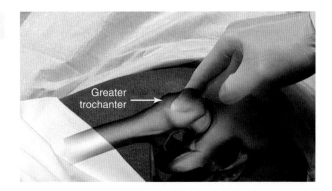

FIGURE 48-1. Trochanteric bursitis.

Greater
trochanter

EQUIPMENT

The equipment includes sterile gloves, povidone-iodine wipes or alcohol wipes, a 22-gauge, 1½- to 2-in. needle and a 5-cc syringe, 1% lidocaine without epinephrine, 20 to 40 mg of methylprednisolone acetate or the equivalent, and an adhesive bandage dressing (Figure 48-2).

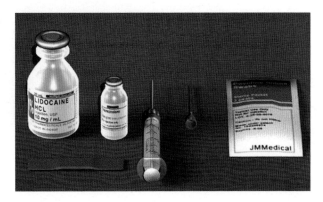

FIGURE 48-2. Equipment.

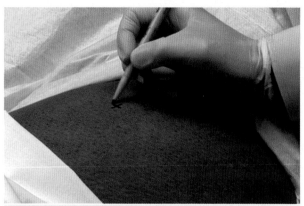

FIGURE 48-3. Mark spot with an indelible marker.

KEY STEPS

1. **Prepare the patient:** Inform the patient of the risks, benefits, and possible complications of injection therapy. Place the patient in a comfortable position on the examining table, and drape the area, leaving the lateral hip exposed. Carefully palpate the lateral thigh. Find the point of maximal tenderness over the prominence of the greater trochanter. Identify the site of entry, and mark it with a thumbnail, ballpoint pen, or indelible marker (Figure 48-3). Prep the area with alcohol or povidone-iodine (Figure 48-4).

2. **Prepare the injection:** Draw up 3 to 5 cc of 1% lidocaine and 20 mg of methylprednisolone acetate or the equivalent into a single syringe, and mix well by tipping the syringe backward and forward. Use a 22-gauge, 1½- to 2-in. needle for the injection.

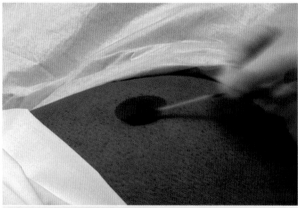

FIGURE 48-4. Prepare the injection site.

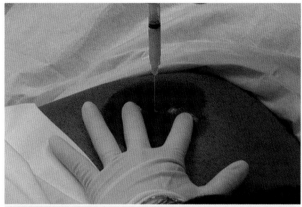

FIGURE 48-5. Inject into the bursa.

3. **Inject the bursa:** Direct the needle perpendicularly to the femur at the point of maximal tenderness, and insert it until bone is felt. Then withdraw the needle 2 to 3 mm (Figure 48-5). After insertion but before injection, pull back the plunger to make sure that the needle is not in a blood vessel. Inject the solution into the bursa.

4. **Massage the bursa:** If the patient is still experiencing discomfort 5 minutes after injection of the bursa and massage of the area, a more distal injection may be necessary at the areas of tenderness (Figure 48-6).

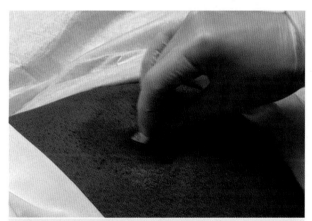

FIGURE 48-6. Massage gently after the injection.

ICD-9 CODES

274.0   Gouty arthropathy
729.5   Leg pain
726.5   Trochanteric bursitis
727.3   Bursitis

Chapter 49

Knee Injection

COMMON INDICATIONS

The knee injection of steroids is a treatment for symptoms of osteoarthritis or inflammatory arthritis of the knee joint (Figure 49-1). As with all joint injections, sterility must be maintained for any components used in the injection that enter the knee-joint space. Knee effusions can be found in several conditions, including septic arthritis. Do not inject steroids into a potentially infected knee.

EQUIPMENT

The equipment for a knee injection includes gloves, povidone-iodine wipes or alcohol wipes, an, 18-gauge needle and a 27-guage, 1½-in. needle, a 3cc syringe, 0.5% Marcaine, 20 to 40 mg of methylprednisolone acetate or its equivalent, and an adhesive bandage dressing (Figure 49-2).

KEY STEPS

1. Draw up 2 cc of Marcaine and 40 mg of methylprednisolone acetate or its equivalent into a syringe using an 18-gauge needle, and mix well by tipping the syringe backward and forward (Figure 49-3).

2. There are three commonly used approaches to knee injections. The upper lateral approach is used if an effusion is present and the removal of fluid is done at the same time as steroids are injected.

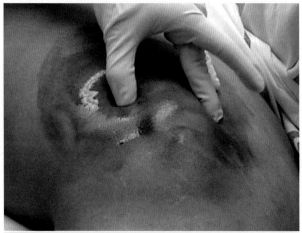

FIGURE 49-1. Osteoarthritis of the knee.

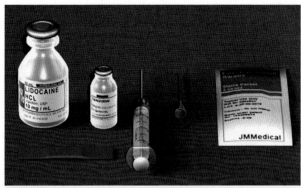

FIGURE 49-2. Equipment.

3. With antiseptic solution, thoroughly clean the skin overlying the knee (Figure 49-4). To perform the injection with the upper lateral approach, place the patient in the supine position with the knee in 20° of flexion. Carefully palpate the knee to identify the anatomic landmarks, including the patella. Assess the size of the effusion, if any (Figure 49-5).

4. Palpate the planned injection site, and mark the site with skin marker or a pen tip (Figure 49-6).

5. Pass the needle through the skin into the knee-joint space so that at least 1 in. of the needle is in the joint space. The needle should be directed under the patella but should not make contact with the underside of the patella. Inject the corticosteroid solution into the joint space. There should be no resistance to the needle tip within the joint itself (Figure 49-7).

6. Withdraw the needle, and apply gentle pressure to the entry site (Figure 49-8).

7. Cover the injection site with an adhesive bandage.

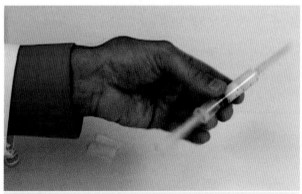

FIGURE 49-3. Draw up the corticosteroid mixture.

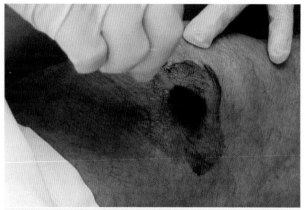

FIGURE 49-4. Prepare the injection site.

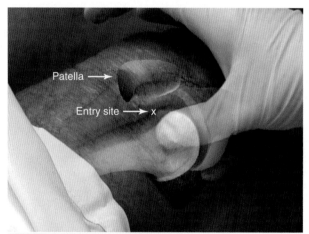

Patella

Entry site → x

FIGURE 49-5. Palpate the joint.

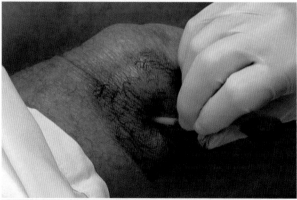

FIGURE 49-6. Mark the entry point.

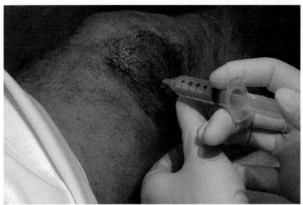

FIGURE 49-7. Inject posteriorly to the patella into the joint space.

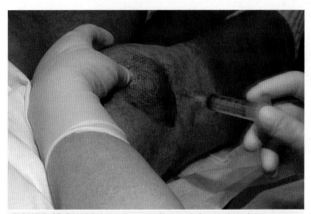

FIGURE 49-8. Withdraw the needle, and dress the site.

ICD-9 CODES

274.0   Gouty arthropathy
696.0   Psoriatic arthritis
714.0   Rheumatoid arthritis
715.16   Degenerative joint disease (DJD) knee
729.5   Leg pain
719.45   Knee pain
719.56   Knee stiffness

Chapter 50

Arthrocentesis

COMMON INDICATIONS

Arthrocentesis allows the sampling or removal of joint fluid and can provide relief to persistent painful effusions. In chronic, degenerative effusions of the knee, a steroid injection can be performed after the aspiration of the joint effusion to relieve pain (Figure 50-1).

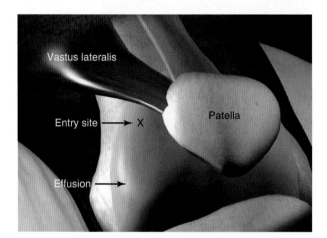

FIGURE 50-1. Anatomy.

Vastus lateralis

Patella

Entry site ⟶ X

Effusion ⟶

EQUIPMENT

The equipment needed for arthrocentesis consists of a large aspiration syringe, lidocaine for anesthetizing the aspiration needle tract, and 0.5% bupivacaine for intra-articular injection if a steroid injection is planned. A 1½ in., 18-gauge needle and a 1½ in., 27-gauge needle are used in combination to draw up and to inject the anesthetic. Two 3-cc syringes are used, one for the block and one for the steroid injection. A sterile preparation and field must be maintained for this procedure (Figure 50-2).

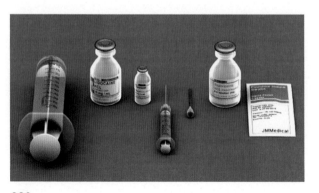

FIGURE 50-2. Equipment.

KEY STEPS

1. **Preparation:** Place the patient in the supine position and with the knee placed in 20° of flexion. Place a towel roll under the knee to support it in flexion. Cleanse the skin with antiseptic solution. Identify the patella and the effusion size by palpation. When aspirating effusions, the ideal location to enter the synovial sac is in the upper outer quadrant of the knee-joint space (Figure 50-3).

Safety tip: Maintain a sterile field and instruments at all times to avoid contamination of the joint space.

2. **Anesthesia:** Inject the local anesthetic along the planned trajectory of the arthrocentesis to reduce the pain of passing the 18-gauge needle through the joint sac. An assistant can hold the syringe and needle in place after the block is injected to act as a visual guide for the passage of the aspiration needle (Figure 50-4).

3. **Aspiration of the fluid:** Pass the 18-gauge needle through the skin along the anesthetized track and into the palpable effusion. The opposite hand compresses the medial aspect of the knee joint to push the intra-articular fluid toward the needle. When the space is entered, withdraw the desired amount of fluid. For tense effusions, withdrawing larger volumes of fluid, up to 50 cc at a time, can reduce pain and improve range of motion (Figure 50-5).

4. **Injection of the steroid (optional):** After the desired amount of fluid is obtained, remove the large syringe from the 18-gauge needle, and replace it with a syringe that is preloaded

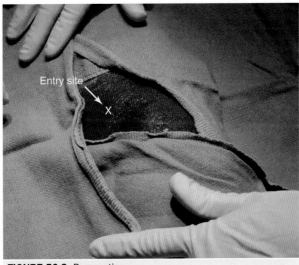

FIGURE 50-3. Preparation.

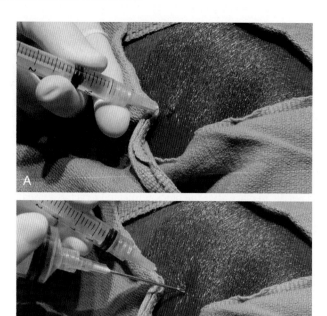

FIGURE 50-4. A-B. Local anesthetic along the trajectory of the aspiration needle.

with 40 mg of triamcinolone or its equivalent. Inject the steroid into the joint space, and withdraw the needle and syringe (Figure 50-6).

Safety tip: Do not inject into tendons or bone. The solution should flow easily into the joint space.

5. **Dressing:** Cover the wound with a sterile bandage.

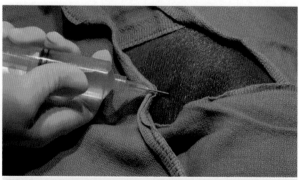

FIGURE 50-5. Aspiration of the effusion.

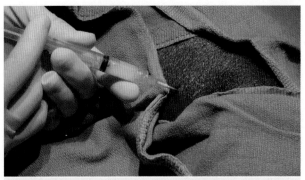

FIGURE 50-6. Steroid injection (if indicated).

ICD-9 CODES

274.0   Gouty arthropathy
696.0   Psoriatic arthritis
714.0   Rheumatoid arthritis
715.16   Degenerative joint disease (DJD) knee
729.5   Leg pain
719.45   Knee pain
719.56   Knee stiffness
726.61   Pes anserine bursitis
727.3   Bursitis
727.51   Baker's cyst

Chapter 51

Trigger Point Injection

COMMON INDICATIONS

Painful trigger points of the low back can be easily injected with a combination of local anesthetics and steroids to obtain immediate and long-term pain relief. Trigger points are commonly found over the sacroiliac joint region where the small ligaments and muscles of the sacrum cross over the iliac crest (Figure 51-1).

EQUIPMENT

For this injection, prepare a 3-cc syringe with 1 cc of bupivacaine, 1.5 cc of lidocaine, and the equivalent of 25 mg of hydrocortisone or 10 mg of triamcinolone. Use an 18-gauge needle to draw up the solutions, but inject with a 25- or 27-gauge needle only (Figure 51-2).

KEY STEPS

1. **Preparation:** Precisely locate the trigger point by firm palpation, using the flat part of the thumb. Cleanse the skin with alcohol (Figure 51-3).

Common trigger point regions

FIGURE 51-1. Anatomy.

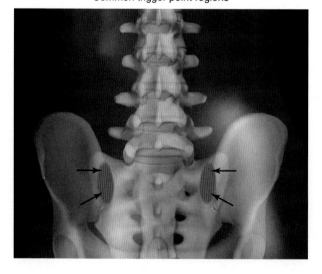

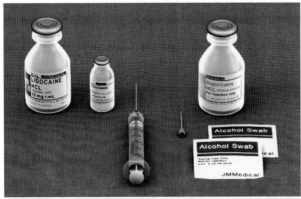

FIGURE 51-2. Equipment.

2. **Injection:** Insert the needle into the center of the palpable trigger point. Inject 0.5 cc of the solution into the center of the trigger point, then inject 0.5 cc into four quadrants within 1 cm of the center of the trigger point. Between each injection, withdraw the needle to a level just below the skin, before repositioning the needle, to ensure that the needle is truly redirected to the different aspects of the trigger point area (Figure 51-4).

3. **Aftercare:** After the injection is complete, massage the solution into the surrounding soft tissue, and obtain feedback from the patient as the local anesthetics take effect. If only partial relief is noted in 5 minutes, a second block can be performed in the area that is still tender. Cover the injection site with a sterile bandage.

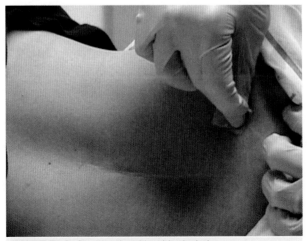

FIGURE 51-3. Cleanse the skin with alcohol.

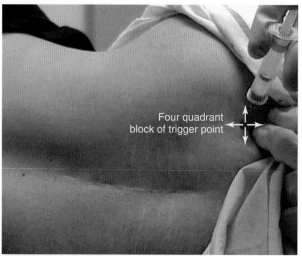

Four quadrant
block of trigger point

FIGURE 51-4. Central and four-quadrant block of the trigger point.

ICD-9 CODES

729.1   Myalgia and myositis, unspecified
723.1   Cervicalgia
723.9   Unspecified musculoskeletal disorders and symptoms referable to neck
724.1   Pain in thoracic spine
724.2   Lumbago
726.19 Other specified disorders (of rotator cuff syndrome of shoulder)

Chapter 52

Shoulder Dislocation Reduction

COMMON INDICATIONS

Shoulder dislocation is a common injury in sports or activities that involve high-velocity injuries such as skiing or contact sports. The most common injury is the anteroinferior dislocation (Figure 52-1). Reduction of this injury in the acute setting improves patient comfort and reduces the risk of neurovascular injury. The patient presents in acute pain, often holding the affected side in flexion and internal rotation. If appropriate monitoring is available, sedation can be useful to provide better muscular relaxation and patient comfort. However, the longer that the dislocation is in place, the greater the spasm that develops. Reduction can be accomplished without sedation in many cases.

TECHNIQUES

There are several methods to reduce the dislocation. The general principle is to apply traction and rotate the humerus externally with a slight extension of the humerus to dislodge it from the inferior aspect of the glenoid fossa (Figure 52-2). In patients with poor muscular development, a simple external rotation or extension may be enough to relocate the shoulder. Scapular

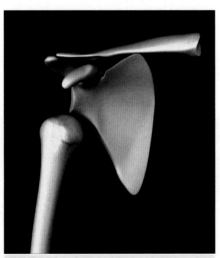

FIGURE 52-1. Anterior-inferior shoulder dislocation.

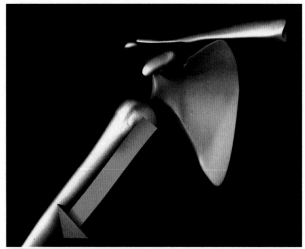

FIGURE 52-2. Traction-and-rotation technique.

rotation, rotating the glenoid fossa downward toward the dislocated humeral head, may also work in similar patients (Figure 52-3).

In athletic patients, the technique combining steady traction (to fatigue the rotator cuff spasm) and slight external rotation is highly successful.

KEY STEPS

1. **Positioning:** Place the patient supine with a sheet or clothing wrapped under the affected axilla crossing over the chest. An assistant stabilizes the patient's torso with traction (Figure 52-4).

2. **Sedation:** Use of a short-acting benzodiazepine (midazolam, 2 mg IV) is ideal for the mild sedation often needed for this procedure. Be cautious with dosing if concurrent opiate pain medications are used.

3. **Reduction of the shoulder:** Grasp the affected arm with one hand above the wrist and one hand above the elbow and the base of the humerus. Apply gentle traction to the arm at a

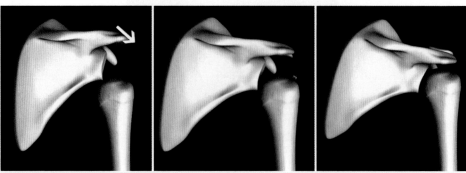

FIGURE 52-3. Scapular-rotation technique.

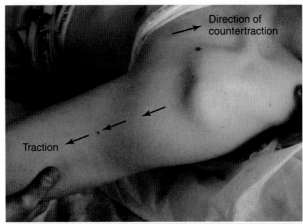

FIGURE 52-4. Direction of countertraction and traction for the traction-rotation technique.

45° angle from the trunk in a slight extension. If crepitus is felt or heard during traction or rotation, stop the procedure, and obtain an X-ray. If there is a history or examination findings that suggest a humeral fracture, do not attempt the relocation before X-rays are obtained. As the deltoid fatigues, gently externally rotate the humerus about 15°. When the muscle is adequately fatigued and the rotation completed, the humerus will relocate back into the glenoid fossa (Figure 52-5).

4. **Splinting of the shoulder:** The patient will note the immediate relief of pain. Hold the arm close to the patient's chest, and place the arm in a sling for 14 days to protect the shoulder from a repeat dislocation. All patients should have rehabilitation for the shoulder to prevent the recurrence of the dislocation.

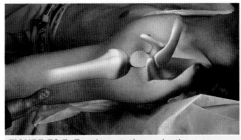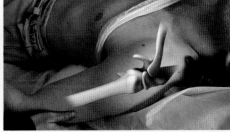

FIGURE 52-5. Traction-rotation reduction.

ICD-9 CODES

2010 ICD-9-CM Diagnosis Code 831.01
Closed anterior dislocation of humerus
2010 ICD-9-CM Diagnosis Code 831.03
Closed inferior dislocation of humerus

INDEX

Note: Page numbers followed by *f* indicate figures.

3